S0-BMR-626

NURSING CASE MANAGEMENT:
From Concept to Evaluation

RT90.7
C64
1993

NURSING CASE MANAGEMENT:

From Concept to Evaluation

Elaine L. Cohen, EdD, RN
Assistant Vice President for Nursing
The General Hospital Center at Passaic
Passaic, New Jersey

Toni G. Cesta, PhD, RN
Director of Nursing for Managed Care
Beth Israel Medical Center
New York, New York

Illustrated

DISCARDED
URI LIBRARY

Mosby

St. Louis Baltimore Boston Chicago London Philadelphia Sydney Toronto

27385648

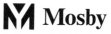

Dedicated to Publishing Excellence

Executive Editor: N. Darlene Como
Associate Developmental Editor: Brigitte Pocta
Project Manager: Mark Spann
Production Editor: Amy Wastalu
Designer: David Zielinski

FIRST EDITION

Copyright © 1993 by Mosby-Year Book, Inc.

All rights reserved. No part of this publication may be reproduced, stored in a retrieval system, or transmitted, in any form or by any means, electronic, mechanical, photocopying, recording, or otherwise, without prior written permission from the publisher.

Permission to photocopy or reproduce solely for internal or personal use is permitted for libraries or other users registered with the Copyright Clearance Center, provided that the base fee of $4.00 per chapter plus $.10 per page is paid directly to the Copyright Clearance Center, 27 Congress Street, Salem, MA 01970. This consent does not extend to other kinds of copying, such as copying for general distribution, for advertising or promotional purposes, for creating new collected works, or for resale.

Printed in the United States of America

Mosby–Year Book, Inc.
11830 Westline Industrial Drive
St. Louis, Missouri 63146

Library of Congress Cataloging in Publication Data

Cohen, Elaine L. (Elaine Liebman)
    Nursing case management :   from concept to evaluation   /   Elaine L. Cohen, Toni G. Cesta. — 1st ed.
        p.   cm.
    Includes bibliographical references and index.
ISBN 0-8016-6698-8
    1. Primary nursing.   I. Cesta, Toni G.   II. Title.
[DNLM: 1. Managed Care Programs—organization & administration.
2. Managed Care Programs—economics.   3. Program Evaluation—methods.   W 125 C678n 1993]
RT90.7.C64   1993
362.1'73—dc20
DNLM/DLC
    for Library of Congress   93-18059
                                                                          CIP

93 94 95 96 97 GW/MV 9 8 7 6 5 4 3 2 1

Dedication

This book is dedicated to all the pioneers and their efforts in the development, research, and evaluation of nursing case management.

Foreword

Writing the first comprehensive text on nursing case management must be recognized for what it is, an awe-inspiring and potentially dangerous undertaking. Nursing case management is evolving moment by moment, not year by year. Its potential to right the ills of health and managed care is well-recognized, but there is little agreement on key issues like definition, scope, or content. In spite of this state of affairs, or because of it, nursing case management arouses considerable passion. For many, myself included, nursing case management is the embodiment of professional nursing practice for today and tomorrow. All potential authors tread lightly when they make any pronouncements about what case management is and what it is not. There will be many readers pleased, but many more who will prepare to go to battle to defend their cherished views and hopes. This is the state of nursing case management today.

Elaine Cohen and Toni Cesta are courageous people. They understood that in order for nursing case management to respond to the growing issues facing health care today, it is essential to bring the core issues of this approach to the table for debate. To ensure a future for nursing case management, we must be able to answer questions, such as: What is the relationship between nursing case management and professional nursing practice? How do we align acute and chronic care models of case management? What difference does the practice of nursing case management make in both quality and cost of health care? Why nurses as case managers?

This book represents a milestone in the history of nursing case management. Its presence indicates that discussion and publications on nursing case management have reached a critical mass where it is now time to look at the whole of the system, where it fits in the evolution of nursing care delivery models, and where it is going. By bringing together current ideas on nursing case management practice, education and research, Cohen and Cesta have offered us an important opportunity to participate in the future of this innovative care delivery model.

Gerri S. Lamb, RN, PhD
Clinical Director for Research
Carondelet St. Mary's Hospital
& Health Center
Tucson, Arizona

Preface

Increasing cost constraints in health care have focused attention on developing and implementing alternative systems of delivering patient care and have stimulated the promotion of national initiatives directed by the Department of Health and Human Services, and supported by the National Commission on Nursing. The purpose of these efforts is to decrease patient length of stay, reduce costs, and improve the quality of patient care.

Hampered by cost containment and quality issues, health care institutions have begun to look at the case management model as a means of improving patient outcomes while controlling costs. The changes in practice patterns associated with nursing case management have helped to reduce costs related to hospitalization.

The basic principles of case management have universal appeal and can be applied to almost any health care setting. Recently attention is being focused on the application of these principles, in particular, the planning, implementation, and evaluation processes.

Nursing Case Management: From Concept to Evaluation is the first book to provide comprehensive data and insights regarding case management as a nursing care delivery system and interdisciplinary model relevant for many health care institutions. It addresses case management primarily from an inpatient perspective. However, examples of the model are provided in a variety of clinical settings. This book also examines what health care providers need to know when implementing case management to contain inpatient expenditures while providing quality patient care. Because evaluation is an integral part of the case management model, this book provides the reader with actual "how to" guidelines for evaluating the factors in nursing case management necessary for meeting the economic and quality-related goals of the organization, direct patient-care providers, and consumers.

This book is written for professionals in clinical and academic health care institutions including administrators, nurses, educators, and students. Discussion moves from a retrospective review of nursing case management to a prospective view for program planning and evaluation.

The book offers the health care professional an informative guide on how to assess the organization and the efficacy of employing nursing case management within the organization. Included are examples for a comprehensive plan to effect the desired change, identifying implementation strategies, and evaluating the clinical outcome of the change process.

The book presents a historical perspective on case management and explains the specific cost-containment issues related to the model. It describes the effect of nursing research on the choice of delivery models for patient care and offers specific methods for evaluating a case management model through data collection and analysis.

The socioeconomic implications of the case management model are discussed and recent policy and legislation issues are analyzed to determine the consequences for future policy development and reform and redesign of patient care. In addition the book provides a detailed analysis of staff education needs and the development of functional roles within the model's framework.

Nursing case management compels us to measure our present practice in relation to the changing health care environment. Applying changes in our practice to the critical issues facing the nursing profession and to influence health care decisions is essential to creating our preferred future.

Nursing case management challenges us to rethink and restructure health care in order to devise effective nursing practice systems and care delivery models. It links nursing education with nursing practices and defines nursing's role in contemporary health care systems. It also plays a crucial role in influencing curricula development for future health care programs.

Rogers (personal communication, 1992) states:

> What we are talking about here is the impact that nursing, given the right milieu, can have on the cost and quality of health care—and it is significant. As nursing case management models are showing, professional nurses—the generalists in health care—are uniquely qualified to perform assessment, monitoring, coordinating, and collaboration functions, as well as traditional hands-on tasks.

Nursing Case Management: From Concept to Evaluation offers a broad understanding of the nursing case management model and lays the foundation for future exploration and research. Our hope is to foster and encourage those who are willing to brave the adventures that lie ahead when reshaping nursing practice and health care management.

Together we would like to express our thanks and gratitude to the many individuals who made the publication of this book possible. Our thanks go to Dr. Judi Haber who introduced us to the staff at Mosby. To our editors, Darlene Como and Brigitte Pocta, for their professional assistance in manuscript development and preparation. To Deborah Forman for her typing services and assistance in meeting deadlines.

To the reviewers, Pamela Becker Weilitz and Mary T. Sinnen, for their valuable comments. A very special thanks is extended to Mike Rogers, a reviewer of the manuscript, who has distinguished himself by his exemplary commitment, effort, support, and thoughtful contributions.

Our deep gratitude goes to Dr. Gerri Lamb for her thought-provoking foreword. Her friendship is truly a gift from the heart. Our appreciation also goes to all the professional nurse case managers who have honored us by sharing their knowledge and expertise.

Our esteem is extended to medical and nursing colleagues for their championship, guidance, and support of collaborative practice.

We also wish to acknowledge our family and friends who through their love and guidance sustained us through the arduous process of writing this book. Our appreciation and indebtedness is expressed to Allan, Pat, Michael, and our parents for their patience and devotion. We are especially indebted to Pat Bushey for her support and invaluable contributions throughout this endeavor.

We would be remiss if we did not acknowledge those individuals who by virtue of their unconditional friendship and sponsorship have influenced our personal and professional growth and success.

To Irene McEachen, Vice President for Nursing, Beth Israel Medical Center, New York, for her vision and risk taking and to Mary Ellen Rauner, Vice President for Nursing, The General Hospital Center at Passaic, for her leadership and guidance. Both have believed in us and accorded us the freedom to pursue our professional dreams.

A personal thank you to Dr. Tricia Munhall for her love, wisdom, and ability to channel energy in all the right directions. And to Dr. Eleanor Lambertsen who continues to be a source of inspiration and creativity.

E.L.C.
T.G.C.

Contents

EVOLUTION OF CASE MANAGEMENT

1

Overview of Health Care Trends

CHAPTER OVERVIEW

Many dramatic changes in the practice and delivery of health services have contributed to the new realities and complexities of the current health care system. This chapter presents nursing as it exists today and shows how the changing health care system and emerging issues have shaped current nursing practices. The chapter also identifies opportunities for innovation and provides an overview of the trends that have led to the development of the nursing case management approach in the delivery of patient care.

This section also discusses the reasons for the success of the nursing case management model in increasing cost-effectiveness, quality of care, and job satisfaction. Included in this discussion are nurse-physician collaborative practice, management of the patient's environment by coordinating and monitoring the appropriate use of patient care resources, monitoring of the patient's length of stay and patient-outcome standards to produce measurements for evaluating cost-effectiveness, and enhanced autonomy and increased decision-making by direct health care providers.

Nursing case management offers the nursing profession an opportunity to define its role in the health care industry and challenges the profession to identify the work that nurses do in terms of its autonomous value to the patient.

THE CHANGING CARE CLIMATE

The present health care system is fraught with complications, constraints, and uncertainty. Major shifts in the practice and delivery of health care have moved dramatically toward the proliferation of scientific and technological services, increasing government regulation, greater market competition, and economic constraints. Additional emerging trends affecting care include the following:

- Rationed and multitiered distribution of health services
- Increased control mechanisms for quality assurance
- Greater emphasis on productivity and efficiency

3

- Increased ethical and legal concerns
- Rising prevalence of the human immunodeficiency virus (HIV) and related infections
- An aging population
- Fragmented and dehumanized patient care.*

These shifts in the health care industry along with the federal government's prospective payment strategies have raised questions about the quality and effectiveness of health care services. Efforts to control spiraling health care costs have changed the economic position of health care organizations and the delivery of patient services in the acute care setting. Restructured reimbursement and finance mechanisms, which are based on diagnosis related groups (DRG), have prompted hospitals to establish tighter financial controls over spending and to limit facility services primarily to the acutely ill.

The concomitant effects of these initiatives on nursing practice have resulted in fewer patient admissions, shortened length of stay, increased patient turnover, increased severity of patient condition and case mix complexity, intensified patient case work loads, and renewed emphasis on nursing productivity and efficient utilization of resources (Buerhaus, 1987; Curran, Minnick, & Moss, 1987; Hartley, 1987; Kramer & Schmalenberg, 1987).

Intensity of Service/Severity of Illness

The increases in severity of illness along with greater patient care requirements have resulted in a significant increase in the demand for professional nursing care services in hospitals and other health care settings (Aiken & Mullinix 1987; Iglehart, 1987; McKibbin, 1990; Secretary's Commission on Nursing, 1988). The need for more nurses to practice in a technologically complex and cost-constrained environment is expected to grow and is indicative of an aging and more acutely ill population with more severe and chronic conditions requiring intense nursing care (McKibbin, 1990). Workload statistics reveal that since the late 1970s, the ratio of registered nurses needed to care for the hospitalized patient population has increased. In 1977 there were 61.4 full-time equivalent nurses (FTE) for every 100 hospitalized patients. In 1988 this number grew to 98.0 FTEs per 100 patients (McKibbin, 1990).

The increase in demand for more intense nursing care services provided by registered nurses in hospitals was brought about by the prospective payment system. Institutional responses to the practice constraints inherent in these governmental rate-setting programs have affected nursing services and the environment in which nurses work. The use of the prospective payment system has resulted in discontent among nursing professionals because of the associated decline in autonomy and control over practice, decreased influence over hospital

---

*Brown & Brown, 1988; Moritz, Hinshaw, & Heinrich, 1989; Mowry & Korpman, 1987; Rosenstein, 1986; Schramm, 1990; Wesbury, 1990.

faction with the quality of care and inadequate compensation and recognition for services provided (Iglehart, 1987; Styles, 1987).

Organizational variables that influence job satisfaction and the rate of turnover in the nursing profession are well represented in health care literature. This growing body of literature offers nursing suggestions on how to cope with the changing health care environment and how to gain control of nursing practices. Many of the profferred solutions focus on increasing economic rewards, appropriating staff mix and skill, and restructuring the work environment.* Emphasis has been placed on fostering nurse involvement in clinical patient care areas and designing better care delivery systems that are more consumer-oriented and meet the needs of the patients (Ethridge, 1987; Fagin, 1987; Porter-O'Grady, 1988a; Strasen, 1991). In addition, collaborative practice models between registered nurses and physicians are recommended for enhancing professional satisfaction and improving patient outcomes.†

Both the original Magnet Hospitals Study (McClure, Poulin, Sovie, & Wandelt, 1983) and a follow-up investigation (Kramer, 1990) identify the factors that enhance professional nursing practice within the hospital setting. These factors include maintaining a professional status, having autonomy and control over practice, and upholding quality assurance standards. Nursing care delivery systems based on differentiated practice proved cost effective and provided continuity of care and effective resource utilization. In addition, the interprofessional collaborative relationships associated with differentiated practice had a significant effect on job satisfaction, recruitment, and retention of a professional nursing staff. Nursing care delivery systems based on differentiated practice were later shown to contribute to a hospital's overall productivity and fiscal viability (Cohen, 1991; Ethridge & Lamb, 1989; Fifield, 1988; Sovie, 1984; Tonges, 1989a; 1989b).

Nursing case management, which was introduced in 1985 and is considered an outgrowth of primary nursing, allows for quality care while containing costs. This management style has emerged as the professional practice model that increases nurse involvement in decisions regarding standards of practice, and integrates the cost and quality components of nursing services (Zander, 1985). Nursing case management provides outcome-oriented patient care within an appropriate length of stay, uses appropriate resources based on specific case types, promotes the integration and coordination of clinical services, monitors the use of patient care resources, supports collaborative practice and continuity of care, and enhances patient and provider satisfaction (Ethridge & Lamb, 1989; Henderson & Wallack, 1987; Stetler, 1987; Zander, 1987; Zander, 1988a).

---

*Aiken & Mullinix, 1987; Barry & Gibbons, 1990; Iglehart, 1987; Strasen, 1988; Styles, 1987; Taft & Stearns, 1991.
†Del Togno-Armanasco, Olivas, & Harter, 1989; Ethridge, 1987; Olivas, Del Togno-Armanasco, Erickson, & Harter, 1989a; 1989b; O'Malley, Loverage, & Cummings, 1989; Zander, 1988a.

WHAT IS NURSING CASE MANAGEMENT?

The definition of nursing case management varies depending upon the discipline that employs it, the personnel and staff mix used, and the setting in which the model is implemented. Primarily borrowing principles from managed care systems, nursing case management is an approach that focuses on the coordination, integration, and direct delivery of patient services, and places internal controls on the resources used for care. Such management emphasizes early assessment and intervention, comprehensive care planning, and inclusive service system referrals.

Several health care settings have adopted unique methods of monitoring patient care activity and resource distribution, such as critical paths (a description of patient care requirements in outline form), case management care plans (similar to the standard nursing care plan but adapted to nursing case management outcome standards), and multidisciplinary action plans (MAP).

Nursing case management has been described as within the walls (WTW), which emphasizes case management activities in the acute care hospital setting, and as beyond the walls (BTW), which refers to case management in outpatient and community-based environments as well as Health Maintenance Organization (HMO) arrangements (Ethridge, 1991; Ethridge & Lamb, 1989; Rogers, Riordan, & Swindle, 1991).

However one views it, because nursing case management balances the cost and quality components of nursing service and patient care outcomes, it is successfully evolving into a professional model that is both sensitive and responsive to current practice demands. A more detailed and differential analysis of nursing case management models is provided in following chapters of this book.

WHY NURSING CASE MANAGEMENT?

Current models of nursing care delivery are unable to meet many of the challenges and issues posed by the present health care setting and professional practice. When analyzing current models of patient care and studies on recruitment and retention of professional nurses, problem areas emerge. These care systems are based on traditional industrial models that promote conventional practices and regimented reporting structures. The current nursing care delivery approaches do not articulate the association between nursing interventions and patient outcomes; therefore, they are unable to assess the beneficial effects of clinical nursing services in relation to today's costs and reimbursement systems (O'Malley, 1988a; 1988b; Porter-O'Grady, 1988b; Stevens, 1985). In addition, the current unstable economic environment compels providers of health care services to engage in the restructuring and innovative rethinking of priorities related to the delivery and management of patient care. The focus on different approaches to care delivery has prompted health service institutions to look at alternative delivery systems as a means of improving patient outcomes and controlling costs.

Restructured Reimbursement

The current prospective budgeting process rations reimbursement for direct care costs and the patient's anticipated hospital resource use (Joel, 1984). Because payment is predetermined, no allowance is made for expenses incurred above the reimbursable rate. The major indicator of a hospital's financial performance and predictor of resource consumption in this system is the patient's length of stay (Joel, 1984; Shaffer, 1983).

The concept of managed care within the acute care setting has evolved as an alternative approach by which the directives on patient care are determined by predicted patterns of resource use. The managed care system places emphasis on managing the patient's environment by coordinating and monitoring the appropriate use of resources and is an integral component of the nursing case management model (Cohen, 1991). This model seeks to increase accountability for nursing practice and to reduce costs and fragmentation associated with patient care by establishing a mechanism for the regulation and integration of services over the course of an individual's illness (Henderson & Wallack, 1987; Zander, 1988a).

Assessment criteria related to hospital-based nursing case management must be able to assess quality, while monitoring and evaluating the outcomes of professional practice. The method used demands the following from the provider:
- Independent assessment and adjustment to variations in patients' needs as defined in terms of patient diagnosis, severity level, spiritual, emotional, and family concerns
- Identification and utilization of appropriate health care resources
- Comprehensive monitoring of patient discharge programs to ensure continuous access to care (Ethridge & Lamb, 1989; Zander, 1988b).

The basic principles used in case management have universal application and are widely used by insurers to control escalating health care costs. These principles are also used by providers in acute care settings to contain inpatient expenditures and provide quality patient care (McIntosh, 1987; Ricklefs, 1987).

The findings of research studies indicate that the changes in inpatient nursing practice patterns associated with nursing case management have helped reduce costs related to the hospitalization of defined groups of patients within certain DRG categories (Cohen, 1991; Ethridge & Lamb, 1989; Zander, 1988b). Nursing case management has also had a positive effect on the demand-induced nursing care shortage by reorganizing delivery systems to maximize professional decision-making opportunities for nurses while allowing for continuity of patient care. These changes have promoted cost-effectiveness, allowed nurses to maintain professional autonomy, improved relationships between nurses and physicians, and improved care provider satisfaction (Cohen, 1991; Ethridge & Lamb, 1989; Olivas, Del Togno-Armanasco, Erickson & Harter, 1989a; 1989b; Zander, 1988c).

REFERENCES

Aiken, L., & Mullinix, C. (1987). The nurse shortage: Myth or reality. *The New England Journal of Medicine. 317*(10), 641-645.

Barry, C., & Gibbons, L. (1990). DHHS nursing roundtable: Redesigning patient care delivery. *Nursing Management, 21*(9), 64-66.

Brown, B., & Brown, J. (1988). The third international conference on AIDS: Risk of AIDS in health care workers. *Nursing Management, 19*(3), 33-35.

Buerhaus, P. (1987). Not just another nursing shortage. *Nursing Economics, 5*(6), 267-279.

Cohen, E. (1991). Nursing case management: Does it pay? *Journal of Nursing Administration, 21*(4), 20-25.

Curran, C., Minnick, A., & Moss, J. (1987). Who needs nurses? *American Journal of Nursing, 87*(4), 444-447.

Del Togno-Armanasco, V., Olivas, G., & Harter, S. (1989). Developing an integrated nursing case management model. *Nursing Management, 20*(5), 26-29.

Ethridge, P. (1987). Building successful nursing care delivery systems for the future. In National Commission on Nursing Implementation Project (Ed.), *Post-Conference Papers Second Invitational Conference* (pp. 91-99) Milwaukee: W.K. Kellogg Foundation.

Ethridge P., & Lamb, G. (1989). Professional nursing case management improves quality, access, and costs. *Nursing Management, 20*(3), 30-35.

Ethridge, P. (1991). A nursing HMO: Carondelet St. Mary's experience. *Nursing Management, 22*(7), 22-27.

Fagin, C. (1987). Nurses for the future. *American Journal of Nursing, 87*(12), 1593-1648.

Fifield, F. (1988). What is a productivity-excellent hospital? *Nursing Research, 24*(1), 27-32.

Hartley, S. (1986). Effects of prospective pricing on nursing. *Nursing Economics, 4*(1), 16-18.

Henderson, M.G., & Wallack, S.S. (1987). Evaluating case management for catastrophic illness. *Business and Health, 4*(3), 7-11.

Iglehart, J. (1987). Problems facing the nursing profession. *New England Journal of Medicine, 317*(10), 646-651.

Joel, L. (1984). DRGs and RIMs: Implications for nursing. *Nursing Outlook, 32*(1), 42-49.

Kramer, M., & Schmalenberg, C. (1987). Magnet hospitals talk about the impact of DRGs on nursing care, Part I. *Nursing Management, 18*(9), 38-42.

Kramer, M. (1990). The magnet hospitals, excellence revisited. *Journal of Nursing Administration, 20*(9), 35-44.

McClure, M.L., Poulin, M.A., Sovie, M.D., & Wandelt, M.A. (1983). *Magnet hospitals, attrition and retention of professional nurses.* Kansas City, Mo.: American Nurses Association.

McIntosh, L. (1987). Hospital based case management. *Nursing Economics, 5*(5), 232-236.

McKibbin, R. (1990). *The nursing shortage and the 1990s: Realities and remedies.* Kansas City, Mo.: American Nurses Association.

Moritz, P., Hinshaw, A.S., & Heinrich, J. (1989). Nursing resources and the delivery of patient care: The National Center for Nursing Research perspective. *The Journal of Nursing Administration, 19*(5), 12-17.

Mowry, J., & Korpman, R. (1987). Hospitals, nursing and medicine: The years ahead. *Journal of Nursing Administration, 17*(11), 16-22.

Olivas, G., Del Togno-Armanasco, V., Erickson, J.R., & Harter, S. (1989a). Case management: A bottom-line care delivery model: Part I: The concept. *Journal of Nursing Administration, 19*(11), 16-20.

Olivas, G., Del Togno-Armanasco, V., Erickson, J.R., & Harter, S. (1989b). Case management: A bottom-line care delivery model: Part II: Adaptation of the model. *Journal of Nursing Administration, 19*(12), 12-17.

O'Malley, J. (1988a). Nursing case management, part II: Dimensions of the nurse case manager role. *Aspen's Advisor for Nurse Executives, 3*(6), 7.

O'Malley, J. (1988b). Nursing case management, part III: Implementing case management. *Aspen's Advisor for Nurse Executives, 3*(7), 8-9.

O'Malley, J., Loveridge, C., & Cummings, S. (1989). The new nursing organization. *Nursing Management, 20*(2), 29-32.

Porter-O'Grady, T. (1988a). From process model to outcome models. *Aspen's Advisor for Nurse Executives, 3*(5), 3-4.

Porter-O'Grady, T. (1988b). Restructuring the nursing organization for a consumer-driven marketplace. *Nursing Administration Quarterly, 12*(3), 60-65.

Ricklefs, R. (1987, December 30). Firms turn to case management to bring down health care costs. *Wall Street Journal.*

Rogers, M., Riordan, J., & Swindle, D. (1991). Community-based nursing case management pays off. *Nursing Management, 22*(3), 30-34.

Rosenstein, A. (1986). Hospital closure or survival: Formula for success. *Health Care Management Review, 11*(3), 29-35.

Schaffer, F. (1983). DRGs: History and overview. *Nursing and Health Care, 4*(7), 388-396.

Schramm, C. (1990, January). Healthcare industry problems call for cooperative solutions. *Healthcare Financial Management,* 54-61.

Secretary's Commission on Nursing (1988, December). *Final Report (Volume I).* Washington, D.C.: Department of Health and Human Services.

Sovie, M.D. (1984). The economics of magnetism. *Nursing Economics, 2*(2), 85-92.

Stetler, C.B. (1987). The case manager's role: A preliminary evaluation. *Definition, 2*(3), 1-4.

Stevens, B.J. (1985). *The nurse as executive* (pp. 105-137). Rockville, Md.: Aspen Publication.

Strasen, L. (1988). Designing health delivery systems. *Journal of Nursing Administration, 18*(9), 3-5.

Strasen, L. (1991). Redesigning hospitals around patients and technology. *Nursing Economics, 9*(4), 233-238.

Styles, M. (1987). Nursing today and a vision for the future. *Nursing Economics, 5*(3), 103-106.

Taft, S., & Stearns, J. (1991). Organizational change toward a nursing agenda: A framework from the Strengthening Hospital Nursing Program. *Journal of Nursing Administration, 21*(2), 12-21.

Tonges, M. (1989a). Redesigning hospital nursing practices: The professionally advanced care team (ProAct TM) model, part I. *Journal of Nursing Administration, 19*(7), 31-38.

Tonges, M. (1989b). Redesigning hospital nursing practices: The professionally advanced care team (ProAct TM) model, part II. *Journal of Nursing Administration, 19*(9), 19-22.

Wesbury, S. (1988). The future of health care: Changes and choices. *Nursing Economics, 6*(2), 59-62.

Zander, K. (1985). Second generation primary nursing: A new agenda. *Journal of Nursing Administration, 15*(3), 18-24.

Zander, K. (1987). Nursing case management: A classic. *Definition, 2*(2), 1-3.

Zander, K. (1988a). Managed care within acute care settings: Design and implementation via nursing case management. *Health Care Supervisor, 6*(2), 24-43.

Zander, K. (1988b). Nursing case management: Strategic management of cost and quality outcomes. *Journal of Nursing Administration, 18*(5), 23-30.

Zander, K. (1988c, April 11). Conference held on nursing case management. At Memorial Sloan Kettering Hospital, New York.

2

Historical Perspective of Nursing Care Delivery Models Within the Hospital Setting

CHAPTER OVERVIEW

This chapter reviews the history and theory of various models of professional practice and institutional patient care systems used in today's health care environment. The restructuring of health care delivery systems has become a promising and successful solution in dealing with cost containment, patient care, and quality assurance issues. Benefits include managing the appropriate use of health care and personnel resources; providing effective and efficient patient care through comprehensive assessment, planning, and coordination efforts; promoting opportunities for professional development and growth across all health care disciplines through participatory and collaborative practice models; and meeting the needs of both the provider and recipients of care through integrated networks of health services.

EVOLUTION OF NURSING CARE

A historical perspective will help readers see how professional practice and nursing care delivery models evolved and how some of the methodologies used by previous approaches have contributed to the development of nursing case management today.

Various configurations for the delivery of nursing care have evolved within the rapidly changing health care industry. These changes have paralleled major economic, societal, and demographic trends. Most recently, changes in patient requirements have occurred as a result of imposed economic constraints. At present, patients are being discharged with increased severity of illness levels, and alternative access to care is not always available or affordable (Sovie, 1987). The rise of consumerism, with its emphasis on patient involvement, the advances in

scientific technology, and the change in societal values and expectations all contribute to the multifaceted nature of nursing care delivery systems. Several approaches have emerged to meet specific market demands. These modes of delivery
are defined by patient selection and allocation and assignment systems of personnel (Arndt & Huckabay, 1980; Stevens, 1985).

The case method was one of the earliest staffing assignments developed. It
involved the assignment of the nurse to either one patient or a case load of patients
to provide complete care. Sometimes referred to as private duty, the case method
used a patient-centered approach by giving the professional nurse full responsibility for the care of the patients on an 8-hour basis (Poulin, 1985; Stevens, 1985).
This method, considered the precursor of primary nursing (Poulin, 1985), was
inefficient because only one nurse provided all direct care for the patient.

The functional method required a division of labor according to specific tasks
and was a popular improvement of the case method (Stevens, 1985). The functional model, a task-oriented approach, involved the use of a variety of personnel.
It was regarded as a highly efficient, regimented system and was designed to take
advantage of different levels of caregiver skill (Stevens, 1985). In functional care
the nurse was required to organize and manage a number of given tasks within
a certain time.

The issue associated with the functional approach in nursing care delivery
was the fragmentation that occurred when meeting the needs of both patient and
staff. Components of patient care that were not addressed raised the frustration
levels of both the provider and the patient (Poulin, 1985; Stevens, 1985). The
sole reliance on regimental tasks was one of the functional model's major draw-
backs and resulted in dissatisfaction for both the patient and the nurse. The
functional method also did not offer the opportunity to provide comprehensive,
continuous care. Nursing's use of the functional method was the adaptation of
an industrial mode of practice to a service system (Poulin, 1985; Stevens, 1985).

Team nursing changed the assignment orientation from tasks to patients and
addressed the problems of the functional system (Shukla, 1982; Van Servellen &
Joiner, 1984). For instance, patient care needs that might have been missed in a
functional nursing model could be picked up by the team approach. The team
method was developed in the early 1950s by Dr. Eleanor Lambertsen as a way
to use all nursing personnel with various skill levels, (professional nurses, practical
nurses, and nurses' aides). This approach developed in response to the increased
technology and shortage of professional nurses (Lambertsen, 1958). The system
began to evolve with increased efforts for improving the quality of patient care
by focusing on patient outcomes. The professional nurse had the responsibility
for the delivery of patient care services and the supervision, coordination, and
evaluation of the outcomes of nursing care provided by the team members.

The advantage of team nursing over functional nursing included increased
availability of professional nursing skill for a larger number of patients, greater
continuity of care, increased interaction between nurses and patients, and reduced
amount of time spent by professional staff on nonprofessional tasks. The antic-

ipated outcome of such a system was cost-effective nursing care (Chavigny & Lewis, 1984; Hinshaw, Chance, & Atwood, 1981; Lambertsen, 1958; Shukla, 1984).

The team approach was more than a system for the assignment of personnel. The approach relied heavily upon the education, experience, clinical skill, and values of all staff involved in the care of patients. The specifics of nursing care were delineated in the nursing care plan, which included therapeutic, preventive, and rehabilitative steps. Because the care plan was initiated upon admission and developed throughout the course of the patient's hospitalization is was considered cumulative. The plan served as an evaluative measure of patient care and later was adapted as a standard for nursing practice by the Joint Commission on Accreditation of Healthcare Organizations (JCAHO). Although team nursing increased the professional nurse's responsibility for patient outcomes, the limitation in the team approach was related to a greater complexity of role functions and an inability to fit into existing practice systems.

Primary nursing is a configuration of care that promotes greater professional accountability and autonomy and improves continuity of care. This model picks up where team nursing leaves off by having the individual nurse be responsible for the assessment, planning, coordination, and evaluation of the effectiveness of care for a certain number of patients. Primary nursing encourages collaborative practice and promotes patient advocacy (Dieman, Noble, & Russel, 1984; Halloran, 1983; Poulin, 1985; Zander, 1985).

Primary nursing is viewed as a care-planning system rather than a caregiving one. The focus in this model is on the planning process for comprehensive and individualized delivery of care. The process uses the nursing care plan, which outlines preferred patient outcomes (Dieman, Noble, & Russel, 1984; Stevens, 1985). Nurses are held responsible and accountable for the outcome of patient care during hospitalization. The nurse is also expected to use the nursing process as a framework for administering professional and direct care responsibilities (Halloran, 1983).

Studies have compared the economic and cost-effective variables of primary nursing (Daeffler, 1975; Felton, 1975; Hancock, et al., 1984; Hinshaw, Chance, & Atwood, 1981). These studies report that primary nursing contributes to greater patient and staff satisfaction and is less expensive than team nursing (Daeffler, 1975; Felton, 1975). However, the validity of these studies has been questioned. It appears that the reported cost savings and improvement in the quality of care are a result of the competency levels of the professional staff rather than the structure of primary nursing (Shukla, 1981).

For primary nursing to be effective, compatible support systems, such as unit secretaries, need to be in place to provide for the routine and nonprofessional activities of the care setting. However, because of current budget constraints, increased severity of patient conditions, and shortened length of stay, hospitals have difficulty maintaining this system of care. Initially, the concept of primary nursing required an all-professional nursing staff. However, a mix of nursing service staff skills and competencies is currently being used successfully in many hospitals (Poulin, 1985; Stevens, 1985). As a result, this patient care delivery system is assuming characteristics of other patient care models and is evolving into a prototype that can be adapted to alternative delivery models of nursing care.

PROFESSIONAL PRACTICE AND ALTERNATIVE PATIENT CARE DELIVERY MODELS

The unstable nature of health care economics has made it necessary to focus attention on developing and implementing alternative systems for delivery of patient care. The need to deliver health care effectively and efficiently has stimulated the promotion of national initiatives directed by the Department of Health and Human Services and supported by the National Commission on Nursing. The purpose of these efforts was to decrease length of stay, reduce costs, and improve the quality of patient care (National Commission on Nursing Implementation Project [NCNIP], 1986; Secretary's Commission on Nursing, 1988).

To achieve these goals while maintaining viability, patient care-delivery systems must be sensitive to limited fiscal and resource appropriation. The systems must also incorporate cost-effective standards and establish quality assurance outcomes of professional practice. To date, several professional practice and alternative care delivery models have been successfully developed and implemented. These models have prompted major adjustments in the practice environments of their settings.

Some of the fundamental characteristics of these professional practice and care delivery approaches are the adaptability and receptiveness of the approaches to differentiated and professional competency levels of practice, the reconfiguration of patient care and maximum use of nursing personnel resources, the use of collaborative practice arrangements among nurses, physicians, and other health care workers, the redesigning of the relationship between the providers and recipients of health care to improve patient care outcomes, and the enhancement of the relationship between the providers of patient care and the organizational culture supporting them. A description of some of the current models used in practice follows.

Integrated Competencies of Nurses Model (ICON)

The ICON models I and II are examples of the earliest alternate care delivery approaches blending the professional and education competency levels of staff with the health care needs and requirements of patients (Rotkovich, 1986). The nursing care responsibilities in these models, which were set up as demonstration projects, are differentiated on the basis of the nurse's educational preparation. Head nurses are required to have a master's degree and are responsible for the management and distribution of personnel and resources and overall quality of care delivered on the unit. Nurses with baccalaureate degrees are accountable for the assessment, planning, and evaluation activities of the nursing process. Nurses with associate degrees complement the professional nurse in patient care and carry out nursing decisions. In the ICON I model, licensed practical nurses (LPN), nurses with diplomas, and nursing assistants are excluded from the staffing complement.

Although ICON I is considered the nursing care delivery system for the future, another model, ICON II, has been implemented and is running concurrently to help LPNs and nurses with diplomas or associate degrees make the transition into their respective practice roles (Rotkovich & Smith, 1987). The goal of this model is to assist through in-service programs, continual education, and clinical precepting the grandfathering of the associate degree and diploma nurses into the professional nurse's role and the LPNs into the associate nurse's role. This objective is in line with the profession's broader goal of achieving two entry levels of nursing practice.

Cost effectiveness, quality, and job satisfaction variables are being measured and evaluated on an ongoing basis. At present no data have been published relating the effects of staff mix and competency levels of nursing staff on the productivity and quality of patient care using the ICON I and II models. Information on nursing personnel satisfaction and retention is also needed.

South Dakota Demonstration Project

Another nursing delivery model expanding on the theme of differentiated practice has been developed and implemented at Sioux Valley Hospital in South Dakota. This hospital is one of several institutions participating in a statewide demonstration project. The project demonstration sites consist of a consortium of institutions including representation from the acute care setting, long-term care (nursing home), and home health agencies (Koerner, Bunkers, Nelson, & Santema, 1989).

This project, directed by Peggy Primm and sponsored by the Midwest Alliance in Nursing (MAIN), not only differentiates practice at the registered nurse level, it also uses these levels of competencies with a case management delivery system of care. Differentiated job descriptions (developed by MAIN) based on baccalaureate and associate degree nursing competencies have been implemented. These descriptions classify the role into the primary and associate nurse positions. "The primary nurse plans care for patients with complex needs from admission through discharge on their unit. The associate nurse provides direct care on a shift-by-shift basis and utilizes Integrated Clinical Pathways to manage patient care. Both groups coordinate resources and discharge planning to facilitate quality patient outcomes and an appropriate length of stay" (Gibson, 1992a; 1992b). Primary nurses at Sioux Valley Hospital are unit-based and one of their duties is to provide phone followup to patients with complex cases. This followup helps evaluate the patient's discharge plan. Most of the primary nurses at Sioux Valley Hospital have Bachelor of Science in nursing degrees.

The nursing role classification process used by Sioux Valley Hospital is based on a factoring method that takes into account each nurse's experience, willingness, motivation, and educational preparation. This process also involves an assessment by the head nurse as well as a self-evaluation. Implementation of the South Dakota project resulted in revised documentation forms that now provide room for nursing diagnosis and assessments of patient care outcomes (Koerner, Bunkers, Nelson, & Santema, 1989).

The Center for Innovation at Sioux Valley Hospital provided funding and administrative support for the creation of the Center for Case Management. The following description of the case management model was provided by S. Jo Gibson, Clinical Nurse Specialist and Project Director for the Center for Case Management.

Recognizing that certain patients require more than episodic hospital care, the Clinical Nurse Specialist (CNS) manages the cases of these select patients on a continuum. The patients are selected on a case-by-case basis and each must exhibit at least one of the following:

- Chronic illness or high-risk pregnancy
- Cognitive or developmental deficit
- Emotional deficit or decreased coping capacity
- Inadequate caregiver or community support
- High probability for physiologic imbalance
- Fixed financial resources
- History of frequent admission patterns

The projected outcomes for case managed patients include:

- High-quality care on a continuum
- Appropriate use of the health care dollar
- Decreased fragmentation of care across many settings
- Decreased readmission rates
- Decreased severity level upon readmission
- Decreased length of stay
- Appropriate use of resources
- Increased interdisciplinary collaboration
- Enhanced community perception
- Patient, family, physician, and nurse satisfaction

Sioux Valley Hospital has 17 CNSs across three nursing divisions including Critical Care, Adult Specialty Care, and Maternal-Child Health. In addition to case managing patients, the CNSs fulfill all of the role components defined by the American Nurse Association: expert clinician, educator, consultant, and researcher.

Referrals for case management come from nurses, physicians, social workers, employers, trust officers, insurance case managers, and families. The CNS works closely with all members of the health care team including the physician, primary nurse, social worker, utilization review nurse, home health nurse, and other community resource contacts to coordinate all necessary services.

Others who contribute to the success of case management include personnel from finance, medical records, data processing, quality assurance, and utilization review. Case management, therefore, pulls together the resources within the hospital to accurately portray a financial and clinical picture (Gibson, 1992a).

Preliminary data have demonstrated an improvement in job satisfaction, a decrease in hospitalization (from one of the demonstration sites), and decreased costs related to managed care from the home health agency affiliated with Sioux Valley Hospital.

Partners in Practice

The partners-in-practice system, defined by Manthey (1989) as a progression from primary nursing, is a partnership established between an experienced senior registered nurse and an individual who supports the nurse as a technical assistant. The technical assistant is assigned to the nurse, not to a case load of patients. Consequently, by delegating tasks to the technical assistant, the registered nurse is able to concentrate on providing professional patient care.

The registered nurse is responsible for defining the role, standards, and nursing care activities. By providing direction and supervision, the registered nurse is also accountable for the overall care delivered in the partnership. An official contract is used to confirm the relationship, and both members are paired on the same time schedule.

This system of care delivery is highly sensitive to unit-based human resource distribution requirements, skill mix, competency levels, and patient care needs. Because of the emphasis placed on the delivery of productive and efficient health care services, the partners-in-practice system can yield substantial benefits. These benefits include savings in overall budget and personnel salary expenditures as a result of reduced turnover rates, decreased use of staffing agencies, and improved management of supplemental nursing resources. The system enhances nursing staff retention by offering opportunities for advanced clinical training and education.

Contract and Group Practice Models

Contract and group practice models have been implemented at Johns Hopkins Hospital, and they focus on building up the relationship among nursing care providers, the organization, and the environments in which they work. The contract model concentrates on promoting job satisfaction and retention by engaging nursing staff in autonomous decision-making related to unit-based staffing levels and coverage, scheduling activities, standards of practice, quality assurance, and peer review (York & Fecteau, 1987). Another characteristic of this model is that it uses primary nursing. The staff benefits from the associated practice arrangements, which include salaried (versus hourly wage) compensation programs.

The group practice model is another innovative system developed for nurse practitioners who work in the emergency department and provide services to a group of patients needing primary health care (York & Fecteau, 1987). This model, which is built upon the same objectives and goals as the contract model, initiates a productivity incentive that compensates nurse practitioners for the amount of care they provided per patient visit. This model calls for creation of an incentive fund that is allocated as patient target volumes are met.

Both these models prove their economic viability and organizational effectiveness by decreasing costs related to staff turnover and sick time, increasing patient visits and admissions, and decreasing length of stay. Reallocation of staff mix, skill, and competency levels leads to greater productivity and better use of the professional nursing staff. Additional gains include increased job satisfaction because of greater continuity of patient care, increased professional responsibility and autonomy, and reciprocal compensation packages.

The Professionally Advanced Care Team Model (ProACT)

The ProACT model was developed at the Robert Wood Johnson University Hospital to meet the demand-induced nursing shortage, differentiated practice, and prospective payment initiatives (Tonges, 1989a; Tonges, 1989b). This model expands the role and professional practice of the registered nurse by establishing two roles for the nurse. The first role is that of the clinical care manager (CCM) and the second is that of primary nurse.

The CCM role requires a nurse with a baccalaureate degree who manages the care for a case load of patients throughout their hospitalization. This position involves managerial, personnel, clinical, and fiscal accountability. Primary nurses, who are graduates of accredited registered-nurse programs, are given responsibility for 24-hour management of patients on the unit and all direct and indirect caregiving activities. They are also accountable for the assessment, planning, and evaluation components of patient care as well as the delegation of tasks to LPNs and nursing assistants providing direct patient care.

This system maximizes primary nursing through the redistribution of support staff and a restructuring of ancillary services at the unit level. Patient care services that could be supported by non-nursing departments, such as housekeeping, dietary, supplies, and pharmacy, are assigned to the appropriate unit personnel. For example, support-service hosts are responsible for hotel-type functions, such as bed-making, and pharmacy technicians are responsible for ordering, obtaining, and preparing medications, among other duties. By placing accountability for nonclinical services on personnel from the respective support departments, nurses are free to provide comprehensive and coordinated patient care.

The traditional reporting structures and organizational processes are altered to adapt to the ProACT model's premise of restructuring care with the patient as the central focus. Luckenbill & Tonges (1990) reported in a preliminary evaluation that job satisfaction increased through collaborative care efforts among nurses, physicians, and other health care workers and through a well-coordinated support-service system for staff and patients. Additional findings included a 10% decrease in length of stay with specific DRG patients and a concomitant increase in patient revenues that are attributable to nursing interventions.

Mercy Health Services Consortium

A major restructuring of nursing services was initiated by 15 institutions within the Mercy Health Service System. This 3-year effort was in response to a grant from the Robert Wood Johnson/Pew Charitable Trusts titled "Strengthening

Hospital Nursing: A Program to Improve Patient Care." Demonstration project sites included acute care hospitals and long-term and home-care settings (Beyers, 1991; Porter, 1991).

The goal of this project was to restructure nursing services to meet the challenges presented by cost, quality, and health care provider satisfaction (Beyers, 1991). Various models of patient care delivery were adapted for multi-disciplinary involvement in planning and delivery of health care, collaborative relationships between nurses, nursing accountability and autonomy, patient and family participation in health care, continuous quality improvement, support services for physicians and ancillaries, and systems that are responsive to local community needs (Grayson, 1991; Porter, 1991).

Five institutions of the 15 member hospitals were designated to start this project. Two of the five hospitals developed case management delivery models of care, which will be discussed later in the book. The remaining three institutions established a combination of collaborative and dyad-system approaches to nursing practice. These health care innovations are highlighted in the following section.

The Catherine McAuley Health System, Ann Arbor Project. This system is a collaborative practice model that was developed to focus on the coordination and planning of services for patients requiring a wide range of medical, social, and psychiatric interventions and care. The patient population consisted of elderly, indigent, chronically ill, and chemically dependent individuals (Hill & Reynolds, 1991).

A designated unit was established within the institution to reduce the fragmentation and meet the health care needs of these patients. A collaborative practice group was also developed and consisted of registered nurses, physicians, social workers, nutritionists, pharmacists, and financial counselors among others. In keeping with the project's goal of maintaining continuous quality care, the responsibilities of this practice group were extended to include services in an outpatient setting. Evaluation data are not yet available.

The Marion Health Center, Sioux City Project. The Sioux City project involved the restructuring of nursing practice and health care delivery on a medical-surgical inpatient unit (Welte, 1991). The project incorporated a collaborative practice arrangement and the reassignment of ancillary staff to assist in the delivery of patient care. The overall design also incorporated a shared governance model.

Changes in nursing practice were realized as programs were developed to reevaluate role functions and support systems for the unit and pre-hospitalization assessment and evaluation processes, develop information and documentation systems to enhance overall delivery and quality patient care, and promote nurse-patient partnerships.

The Saint Joseph Mercy Hospital, Mason City Project. The Mason City project involved development of a dyad model of nursing practice used on an inpatient oncology unit. This approach outlined role functions for the registered nurse, licensed practical nurse, and nursing assistant. Clinical nurse specialists provided overall leadership and management of patient care.

The main goal of this project was to provide continuous, holistic care in a network of hospital-based units and outpatient, hospice, and community resource settings (Schumacher, 1991). Joint planning committees for nurses and physicians promoted collaboration on health care decisions and evaluated outcomes of patient care. Patient and family support groups provided for many housing, educational, and pastoral needs. Again, the data from this project are not yet available.

NURSING CASE MANAGEMENT

A review of the literature indicates that aspects of some of the past and current nursing practice approaches and delivery models of care were incorporated into the development of nursing case management. The strength of nursing case management comes from the philosophy and collaborative practice strategies of both primary and team nursing. In fact, some of the care planning and coordination processes used in these models are reflected in the critical paths and care plans of nursing case management. These plans are used to monitor patient care requirements and activity as well as the resources for meeting those needs.

With former models, nursing care revolved around the nursing care plan, which provided a broad-based outline for the delivery of nursing services for the patient. These plans gave little direction in establishing a structure for achieving expected outcomes of nursing care for each day of hospitalization. The nursing case management model, however, provides a framework for nurses to manage the patient's hospital stay. Directing the delivery of patient care services allows the nurse to anticipate needs, thereby providing the opportunity for overall coordination and integration of outcomes and cost (Cohen & Cesta, 1992; Zander, 1990).

Nursing case management also integrates many of the professional practice demands and initiatives characteristic of alternative patient care delivery models. By emphasizing care that is patient-centered, the nursing case management approach embraces techniques of business in which the patient is seen as the customer and valuable consumer who has the right to demand the best in health care. Placing the patient at the core of nursing's power base authorizes the profession to reconfirm its commitment to society. Nursing case management incorporates a new way of looking at the relationships among cost, quality, and nursing care. It places an emphasis on the autonomy, authority, and accountability of professional nursing practice by promoting an open system of care in which information is shared among all disciplines. The individual method of providing patient care is replaced by a team whose members work collaboratively (Cohen & Cesta, 1992). Because of its universal applicability, an in-depth discussion and treatment of the nursing case management model will be provided in Unit II.

REFERENCES

Arndt, C., & Huckabay, L. (1980). *Nursing administration theory for practice with a system approach* (pp. 65-111). Chicago, Illinois: American Hospital Association.

Beyers, M. (1991). Restructuring nursing services in the Mercy Health Services Consortium. *Nursing Administration Quarterly, 15*(4), 43-45.

Chavigny, K., & Lewis, A. (1984). Team or primary nursing care? *Nursing Outlook, 32*(6), 322-327.

Cohen, E., & Cesta, T. (1992). *The economics of health care and the realities of nursing in the 1990s.* Manuscript submitted for publication.

Daeffler, R.J. (1975). Patient's perception of care under team or primary nursing. *Journal of Nursing Administration, 6*(3), 20-26.

Dieman, P.A., Noble, E., & Russel, M.E. (1984). Achieving a professional practice model: How primary nursing can help. *Journal of Nursing Administration, 14*(7), 16-21.

Felton, G. (1975). Increasing the quality of nursing care by introducing the concept of primary nursing: A model project. *Nursing Research, 24*(1), 27-32.

Gibson, S. (1992a). *Center for case management Sioux Valley Hospital.* Unpublished manuscript.

Gibson, S. (1992b). Personal communication.

Grayson, M. (1991, August 5). System uses financial data and grass roots ideas to restructure care delivery. Hospitals, 31-32.

Halloran, E. (1983). Staffing assignment: By task or by patient. *Nursing Management, 14*(8), 16-18.

Hancock, W.N., et al. (1984). A cost and staffing comparison of an all-RN staff and team nursing. *Nursing Administration Quarterly, 8*(2), 45-55.

Hill, B., & Reynolds, M. (1991). The Catherine McAuley Health System, Ann Arbor Project. *Nursing Administration Quarterly, 15*(4), 48-50.

Hinshaw, A.S., Chance, H.C., & Atwood, J. (1981). Staff, patient and cost outcomes of All-RN registered nurse staffing. *Journal of Nursing Administration, 11*(11), 30-36.

Koerner, J.E., Bunkers, L., Nelson, B., & Santema, K. (1989). Implementing differentiated practice: The Sioux Valley Hospital experience. *Journal of Nursing Administration, 19*(2), 13-20.

Lambertsen, E. (1958). *Education for nursing leadership.* Philadelphia: J.B. Lippincott Company.

Luckenbill, J., & Tonges, M. (1990). Restructured patient care delivery: Evaluation of the ProACT TM model. *Nursing Economics, 8*(1), 36-44.

Manthey, M. (1989). Practice partnerships: The newest concept in care delivery. *Journal of Nursing Administration, 19*(2), 33-35.

National Commission on Nursing Implementation Project (1986, November 7). *Invitational Conference.* Milwaukee: W.K. Kellogg Foundation.

Porter, A. (1991). The Consortium Demonstration Project planning. *Nursing Administration Quarterly, 15*(4), 45-48.

Poulin, M. (1985). Configuration of nursing practice. In American Nurse's Association (Ed.), *Issues in professional nursing practice* (pp. 1-14). Kansas City, Mo.: The Association.

Rotkovich, R. (1986). ICON: A model of nursing practice for the future. *Nursing Management, 17*(6), 54-56.

Rotkovich, R., & Smith, C. (1987). ICON I—The future model, ICON II—The transition model. *Nursing Management, 18*(11), 91-96.

Schumacher, L. (1991). The St. Joseph Mercy Hospital, Mason City Project. *Nursing Administration Quarterly, 15*(4), 56-58.

Secretary's Commission on Nursing (1988, December). *Final Report (Volume I).* Washington, D.C.: Department of Health and Human Services.

Shukla, R.K. (1981). Structure vs. people in primary nursing: An inquiry. *Nursing Research, 30*(7), 236-241.

Shukla, R.K. (1982). Primary or team nursing? Two conditions determine the choice. *Journal of Nursing Administration, 12*(11), 12-15.

Shukla, R.K., & Turner, W.E. (1984). Patient's perception of care under primary and team nursing. *Research in Nursing and Health, 7*(2), 93-99.

Sovie, M.D. (1987). Exceptional executive leadership shapes nursing's future. *Nursing Economics, 5*(1), 13-20.

Stevens, B.J. (1985). *The nurse as executive* (pp. 105-137). Rockville, Md.: Aspen Publication.

Tonges, M. (1989a). Redesigning hospital nursing practice: The professionally advanced care team (ProACT℠) model, part I. *Journal of Nursing Administration, 19*(7), 31-38.

Tonges, M. (1989b). Redesigning hospital nursing practice: The professionally advanced care team (ProACT℠) model, part II. *Journal of Nursing Administration, 19*(9), 19-22.

Van Servellen, G.M., & Joiner, C. (1984). Convergence among primary nurses in their perception of their nursing functions. *Nursing and Health Care, 5*(4), 213-217.

Welte, V. (1991). The Marian Health Center, Sioux City Project. *Nursing Administration Quarterly, 15*(4), 54-56.

York, C., & Fecteau, D. (1987). Innovative models of professional nursing practice. *Nursing Economics, 5*(4), 162-166.

Zander, K. (1985). Second generation primary nursing: A new agenda. *Journal of Nursing Administration, 15*(3), 18-24.

Zander, K. (1990). Managed care and nursing case management. In G.G. Mayer, M.J. Madden, & E. Lawrenz (ed.), *Patient care delivery model,* (pp. 37-61). Rockville, Md.: Aspen Publishers, Inc.

3

Historical Development of Case Management

CHAPTER OVERVIEW

The case management approach represents an innovative response to the demands of providing care in the least expensive setting and coordinating and planning for needed community resources. For the past 20 years there has been a growth in the variety of case management delivery systems of care.

This chapter reviews the historical development of the case management concept. Descriptions of different non-nursing case management models are given to make the reader aware of the vastness and complexity of this approach. This is not intended to suggest limited use of the case management model. On the contrary, its great potential and applicability should be promoted. Studies show that this model can be an effective and efficient system by focusing on and caring for the health and social needs of the individual.

INTRODUCTION OF CASE MANAGEMENT

Most of the literature on nursing case management practiced in the acute care setting is new. However, case management has been used by mental health and social services for years. For more than two decades, the case management approach has been used as an alternate design for the delivery of health care. The first federally funded demonstration project began in 1971 and has been associated with a number of methods to coordinate and provide comprehensive services of care for the individual (Merrill, 1985). Regardless of the different approaches, the main principle underlying case management is ensuring the quality as well as the efficiency and cost-effectiveness of services provided (Weil & Karls, 1985). Emphasis is placed on the recipient of case managed care and the coordination and networking of services (Weil & Karls, 1985; White, 1986).

Research related to the outpatient and community-based population has studied the effects of health care case management, in areas other than nursing. The specific target groups included the frail elderly, the chronically ill who are functionally or emotionally challenged, and clients who require long-term care services. These case management projects were designed to use less expensive, community-based services in order to prevent unnecessary institutionalization (Steinberg & Carter, 1983; Zawadski, 1983). Various services, from companionship to homemaking, were provided to assist individuals in their daily activities.

Findings of these studies show that case-managed, in-home support services, such as mental health, respite care, and homemaker or personal care services, have been effective in improving access (evidenced by shorter service waiting lists), assessment, and care planning needs of elderly clients (EISEP, 1988; Raschko, 1985). Additional studies illustrate the efficacy of case management in coordinating and integrating health and social services for long-term care, assessing quality-of-life outcomes (quality-of-living conditions), and reducing time spent in long-term care facilities (Carcagno & Kemper, 1988; Eggert, Bowlyow & Nichols, 1980; Sherwood & Morris, 1983).

Because the nursing profession recognizes the need for changes in the system of health care delivery, more and more nurses are being designated as case managers. This change is due to nurses' expertise and knowledge in managing patient care. Case managers are involved in the assessment, coordination, referral, individualized planning, monitoring, and follow-up activities associated with case management (Grau, 1984; Johnson & Grant, 1985; Mudinger, 1984).

Primarily used with long-term care populations, case management arrangements have recently been developed by private insurance carriers as cost-containment strategies, and have also been integrated into the acute care setting (Henderson & Collard, 1988; McIntosh, 1987). Consequently, different models of case management have evolved. Merrill (1985) identified three categories of case management: social, primary care, and medical/social.

SOCIAL CASE MANAGEMENT

Social case management models emphasize comprehensive long-term community care services used to delay hospitalization. Both health and social needs are addressed in this setting. Primarily successful with the elderly population, this model focuses on ensuring the independence of the individual through family and community involvement. It is based on a multidisciplinary approach to coordinate the care of the patient.

A variety of services, from companionship to homemaking, are offered to assist individuals in their daily activities. One example of the social case management approach is the U.S. Department of Housing and Development's Congregate Housing Services Program, in which nonhealth services are provided to the elderly living in a housing project.

PRIMARY CARE CASE MANAGEMENT

Primary care case management takes on the role of gatekeeper based on the medical model of care. This approach focuses on the treatment of a particular health problem and tries to prevent institutionalization. In this model, the physician functions as the case manager and has the responsibility of coordinating services and managing the patient (Johnson & Grant, 1985).

Primary care case management emphasizes the need to regulate resource use to assure cost-effectiveness. Examples mentioned include HMOs, which originally served Medicaid beneficiaries and have become increasingly popular among insurance companies as a means of controlling the disproportionate use of medical care.

Since the patient population accommodated by primary care case management is defined by health status, the type of case management services required varies according to the health needs of the patient. The financial imperatives to curtail high-cost medical technology are strong under the primary care case management system. However, a major liability of this approach is the exclusion of necessary medical services and hospitalization. Johnson and Grant (1985) recommend that quality assurance standards be incorporated into this mode of health care delivery.

MEDICAL/SOCIAL CASE MANAGEMENT

The medical/social case management model focuses on the long-term-care patient population at risk for hospitalization. This model combines available resource utilization with additional services, which are not traditionally covered by health insurance, to maintain the individual in the home or community. The case manager(s) in this system may be drawn from nurses, physicians, social workers, and family members who have input into the assessment, coordination, care planning, and care monitoring.

An example of the medical/social case management model is the social/HMO demonstration project, which integrates both medical and social services on a prepaid capitated basis, to meet the multiple needs of the chronically ill patient. This model emphasizes providing the least restrictive and least costly long-term care by identifying the appropriate services and coordinating its delivery.

Additional definitions of the case management model are offered by White (1986), who bases the case management approach on a continual process of responsibility and authority for the provision of care and resource appropriation and use. Along this spectrum situations arise that either preclude the use of case management or facilitate case management arrangements with direct health service delivery.

Five case management models were also characterized. These models are differentiated on the basis of authority level of the client, support and financial systems, and payment allocation (White, 1986).

1. Restricted market—In this arrangement, the clients become their own case managers and negotiate for services among independent providers.
2. Multiservice agency—This system allows an agency to provide its own health care.
3. Advocacy agency—With this model, some case management is provided along with direct patient care services.
4. Brokerage agency—The agency in this system acts as a broker in coordinating, controlling, and monitoring services and resources.

5. Prepaid long-term-care organization—With this arrangement, a company contracts for case management services and coordinates resources on a prepaid, capitated basis.

Weil (1985) further characterized case management into three practice models: the generalist case manager or broker model, the primary-therapist-as-case-manager model, and the interdisciplinary team model.

The generalist case manager model is structured to provide direct service, access, planning, and monitoring activities to clients. The case manager in this system acts as a broker and is involved in the intake, coordination, and evaluation processes.

A broad range of professional disciplines may be represented; therefore, the case managers in this model may include social workers, nurses, and mental health or rehabilitation specialists. Continuous and efficient service is assured because of the close working relationship between the case manager and client. The case manager also benefits from autonomous decision-making and other independent management responsibilities.

The primary therapist model emphasizes a therapeutic relationship between the case manager and client. The case manager in this system is required to have a master's degree and training in either psychology, social work, psychiatry, or psychiatric clinical nursing specialties.

As in the generalist model, the case manager-patient relationship is a close one with the case manager responsible for coordination and evaluation services. Because of this one-on-one relationship, the primary therapist model works well with small, community-based programs and has been successful in coordinating and planning efforts and resources with larger networking systems.

Initiatives to ensure the delivery of case management are strong under the primary therapist model. However, therapeutic services have been known to take precedence at the expense of case management functions. Weil (1985) recommend the supplementation of case management responsibilities with therapeutic care.

The interdisciplinary team model focuses on providing case management services through a collaborative team approach. The responsibilities and designated case management functions are divided among the team members according to their area of specialization and expertise.

In this system the case managers may include nurses, social workers, or therapists who have accountability and provide services within their own area of concentration. One team member, however, is appointed to maintain overall service coordination and evaluation.

The benefits of the interdisciplinary team approach include improved continuity of care and enhanced coordination of services and staff support systems to promote mutual program-planning, problem-solving, and client advocacy.

PRIVATE CASE MANAGEMENT

Private case management systems have evolved to meet the needs of clients outside publicly funded programs or those who prefer more personalized services

(Parker & Secord 1988). Parker and Secord cite the findings of a major survey conducted by Inter-Study's Center for Aging and Long-Term Care and funded by the Retirement Research Foundation.

This study investigated the characteristics, services, referral and funding sources of private geriatric-case-management firms across the United States. According to Parker and Secord, this model evolved as a result of an increase in the elderly population, escalating health care costs, growing need for integrated social and health services for the elderly, and increasing emphasis placed on long-term care issues. Survey findings are discussed in the following five paragraphs.

Private case management firms were in business an average of 3 years and most (98.9%) were independently owned, run for profit, and self-managed. Some affiliations existed with hospitals, public and private social service agencies, and nursing homes. Clientele consisted of elderly individuals with mean annual incomes ranging from $5,000 to $15,000. Case managers in this system were college graduates who were prepared in social work or nursing and who carried a small case load of clients.

In most instances, private case management functions included coordination of services, social, functional, financial; mental health assessment and counseling; and referral, monitoring, and evaluation services. Medical assessments were done by physicians in 44% of the private case management businesses. Some of the other services consisted of nursing home and housing placement, retirement planning, companion and homemaker services, and transportation and respite care. These direct services were provided more frequently by for-profit and unaffiliated private case management businesses than by the nonprofit and affiliated companies. Those firms that employed registered nurses as case managers had a tendency to provide more direct care services as well.

Services most often referred to by private case managers included home health care, homemaker, and personal care services, family and legal counseling, and physical therapy. Referral sources were composed of physicians, social workers, family members, and self-referrals.

Private case managers were able to provide more individualized services and were also accessible on off hours, weekends, and holidays.

Reimbursement for services provided by private case managers ranged from hourly and set rates per session to service and package rates. Unaffiliated and for-profit businesses used more hourly and set rate methods and also segregated their services to charge for case management functions involving more time and attention. Sliding fee scales were more common in affiliated and nonprofit organizations. Funding sources to private case management businesses included out-of-pocket payments by client and/or family members, private insurance, Medicare, Medicaid, and other sources that consisted of public funds, trusts, and grants.

Benefits of private case management approaches for staff members include increased flexibility and autonomy in decision-making, independent planning and coordinating of services, greater income, and professional satisfaction. Clients and their families also reported improved accessibility to case managers, less duplication and redundancy of services, very individualized care, and long-term association with one case manager. However, further evaluation is needed regarding access to other health care services, overall quality of private case management care, cost, and reimbursement issues.

COMPONENTS OF CASE MANAGEMENT

Weil (1985) extensively outlined the main service components common in all case management models.

Client Identification and Outreach—Individuals who are eligible or need case management services are identified. Admission to a case management program is determined by interview process, referral, and networking systems, or by the case manager actively promoting eligibility for individuals who might not inquire about case management services for themselves (for example, individuals who are indigent or have mental illness).

Individual Assessment and Diagnosis—Case managers use their comprehensive knowledge and skill to assess the physical, emotional, and psychological needs as well as the social and support requirements of their clients. This process aids in the coordination, facilitation, monitoring, and access of case management services.

Service Planning and Resource Identification—With the collaboration of the client, the case manager assumes the responsibility for coordinating and planning care services. This includes the development of care plans and determining resource and networking systems.

Linking Clients to Needed Services—Case managers act as brokers to expedite and follow through with the coordination and planning needs of the client. Both community and agency resources may be used. In some systems, this responsibility involves actually transporting the client to a recommended service.

Service Implementation and Coordination—The case manager ensures that the identified needs are achieved and follows the formal agreements made with the networking agencies. This is done by extensive documentation and record-keeping of the efficiency, effectiveness, and quality of case management care services. A participative relationship of client and case manager and autonomous decision-making on the part of the case manager are crucial to both groups' engagement in the system.

Monitoring service delivery—The case manager is responsible for directing and overseeing the distribution of services to the client. A multidisciplinary and multiservice relationship is promoted to assure appropriate and effective delivery of case-managed services.

Advocacy—Case managers act on behalf of the client in assuring that needed interventions are obtained and that the client is making progress in the program. As explained by Weil, the advocacy strategy is used not only for the individual client but for the benefit of all individuals in common predicaments.

Evaluation—The case manager is responsible and accountable for appraising the specific as well as the overall usefulness and effectiveness of case managed services. The evaluation process involves continuous monitoring and analysis of the needs of the individuals and services provided to the clients. Early identification of changes or problems with the client or the provider of services is made, ensuring timely intervention and replanning by the case manager.

REFERENCES

Carcagno, G.J., & Kemper, P. (1988). The evolution of the National Long Term Care Demonstration: An overview of the Channeling Demonstration and its evaluation. *Health Services Research, 23,* 1-22.

Eggert, G.M., Bowlyow, J.E., & Nichols, C.W. (1980). Gaining control of the long term care system: First returns from Access Experiment. *The Gerontologist, 20,* 356-363.

EISEP (1988, November 30). *An evaluation of New York City's home care services supported under the expanded in-home service for the elderly program.* Health Research: New York University. Funded by New York City's Department for the Aging (contract #11000100).

Grau, L. (1984). Case management and the nurse. *Geriatric Nurse, 5,* 372-375.

Henderson, M.G., & Collard, A. (1988). Measuring quality in medical case management programs. *Quality Review Bulletin, 14*(2), 33-39.

Johnson, C., & Grant, L. (1985). *The nursing home in American society* (pp. 140-200). Baltimore: Johns Hopkins University Press.

McIntosh, L. (1987). Hospital based case management. *Nursing Economics, 5*(5), 232-236.

Merrill, J.C. (1985). Defining case management. *Business and Health, 3*(5-9), 5-9.

Mudinger, M.O. (1984). Community based case: Who will be the case managers? *Nursing Outlook, 32*(6), 294-295.

Parker, M., & Secord, L. (1988). Private geriatric case management: Providers, services and fees. *Nursing Economics, 6*(4), 165-172, 195.

Raschko, R. (1985). Systems integration at the program level: aging and mental health. *The Gerontologist, 25,* 460-463.

Sherwood, S., & Morris, J.N. (1983). The Pennsylvania Domiciliary Care Experiment: Impact on quality life. *American Journal of Public Health, 73,* 646-653.

Steinberg, R.M. & Carter, G.W. (1983). *Case management and the elderly: A handbook for planning and administering programs.* Lexington, Mass.: Lexington Books.

Weil, M., & Karls, J. (1985). Historical origins and recent developments. In M. Weil, & J. Karls (Ed.), *Case management in human service practice* (pp. 1-28). San Francisco: Jossey Bass Publishers.

White, M. (1986). Case management. In G.L. Maddox (Ed.), *The encyclopedia of aging* (pp. 92-96). New York: Springer Publishing.

Zawadski, R.T. (1983). The long-term care demonstration projects: What are they and why they came into being? *Home Health Care Services Quarterly, 4*(3-4), 5-26.

CONTEMPORARY MODELS OF CASE MANAGEMENT

The Difference Between Managed Care and Nursing Case Management

CHAPTER OVERVIEW

As the demand for cost-effective high-quality health care continues to grow, innovative approaches to improving patient care delivery must be explored. These goals can only be achieved within a framework of total organizational commitment to restructuring care to meet the needs of today's health care provider and the present patient population.

Managed care and case management are both effective approaches that can be used in the reorganization process. As discussed, both systems help define the role and scope of the nurse's responsibilities in the delivery setting. These models can enhance the productivity and competency levels of staff by organizing personnel to use their varying skills and expertise in better ways. This could result in increased professionalism and satisfaction of all providers.

By ensuring that appropriate outcomes are achieved, both managed care and case management provide a framework for continuous and refined planning of nursing and multidisciplinary care and ensure appropriate and cost-effective use of patient resources. Finally, these models can contribute to the foundation of total quality improvement and ensure continued delivery of high-quality patient care.

THE MANAGED CARE/CASE MANAGEMENT ALTERNATIVE

Because managed care and case management have been used interchangeably in the professional literature, confusion as to the difference between the two concepts arises. Furthermore, managed care and case management share a common ground in their historical development and have similar purposes and goals relating to cost containment and quality care. These similarities add to the confusion.

Cost management issues and quality care, which at one point were on opposite sides of the health care delivery spectrum, are now being integrated into one system. The economic power that had been reserved for physicians and hospitals has been transferred to the purchasers of health services, which include business corporations, insurance companies, and individuals. The buyers' objectives comprise coordinating and managing the use of health services and allocating resources for future distribution.

Managed care emerged as control shifted from the provider to the purchaser of health services. The managed care system links the provider with the patient to manage costs, access, and quality components of health care delivery. Major health policies like the federal Health Maintenance Organization Act, adopted in the early 1970s, established a trend for the growth of managed care programs. The HMOs and Preferred Provider Organizations (PPO), two popular examples, offered an alternative to costly inpatient care through the provision of cost-effective treatments and multiple preventive and outpatient services.

Case management is used in these managed care plans as a cost-containment initiative. It further grounds the managed care approach by focusing on the individual health care needs of the patient. Case management is effective because it targets the coordination, integration, and outcome evaluation processes of care.

The inherent strengths in both the managed care and case management systems have led to a renewed interest in the utility and effectiveness of such systems. Both systems are currently being used as strategic approaches to the restructuring of the delivery aspects of health care.

DEFINING MANAGED CARE AND NURSING CASE MANAGEMENT

In a traditional context, managed care is viewed as a system that provides the generalized structure and focus when managing the use, cost, quality, and effectiveness of health care services. Managed care then becomes an umbrella for several cost containment initiatives that may involve case management.

On the other hand, nursing case management can be conceptualized as a process model, the underpinnings of which are essential in attending to the many components and services used in the delivery aspects of patient care. The case-managed approach is based upon and includes variations on the managed care theme.

Aside from its broader application, managed care has been further diversified as its principles have been adapted to the inpatient, acute care setting. In this setting, managed care has evolved in its own right into a separate professional nursing care delivery model.

Various definitions have been offered in an attempt to distinguish managed care from nursing case management. Managed care is a nursing care delivery system that supports cost-effective, patient outcome—oriented care. It is unit-based and structurally designed to promote and support care at the patient's bedside. Patient assignments are not targeted to any particular case type, and critical paths and case management care plans are used to ensure support for critical paths and case management care plans are used to ensure support for standardized patterns of care and length of hospitalization for the individual patient. Managed care can also be used with primary, team, functional, and alternative nursing care delivery systems.

Continuous monitoring and evaluating of the patient's care is maintained through interdisciplinary team meetings, and variances from the plan of care are analyzed by the unit's nurse manager or patient care manager (Cesta, 1991; Etheredge, 1989; Zander, 1991).

One of the strengths of the managed care system is that it can be structured to use staff through differentiated practice arrangements and competency levels of nursing personnel. In short, managed care implies a consistency of plan in that what is done to or for a given patient is consistent even though individual care givers may change (Zander, 1991).

Case management differs from managed care in that the accountability and responsibility for the delivery of care is based on an entire occurrence of hospitalization for a targeted DRG group of patients and is not geographically confined to that patient's unit (Etheredge, 1989; Zander, 1990). This widens the circumscribed area of patient services to include patient care planning and coordination across health care settings. Case management, then, implies consistency of provider: even though different, formal, informal, and even very esoteric resources are used, the coordinator or provider (usually an individual) remains the same (Zander, 1991).

Collaborative practice arrangements in the form of group practice are supported, and interdisciplinary decision-making is facilitated to ensure appropriate use of patient resources and achievement of expected clinical outcomes. Collaboration usually includes members of the health care team and the patient or family to help accomplish anticipated care outcomes. Critical paths and case management plans are used by the participants of the health care teams. Variance analysis and evaluation of patient care is expanded beyond the confines of the patient unit and encompasses all patients in the specific case load (Etheredge, 1989; Zander, 1990).

An example of a case management model, called the Beth Israel Case Managed Patient Care Model (Cesta, 1991), was developed for use within an acute care setting. Using the practice concepts of both primary and team nursing, this model supports the coordination and management of the care of patients from admission to discharge. The objectives of the model are as follows:

1. Improve quality of care.
2. Control resource utilization.
3. Decrease length of stay.
4. Increase patient satisfaction.
5. Increase staff satisfaction.

This managed patient care model, which was implemented through a reorganization of the nursing department structure, provides the opportunity for advancement of selected registered nurses working at the patient bedside. Through the use of a managed care career ladder, nurses who have a baccalaureate degree and have demonstrated advanced clinical and leadership skills can remain in the direct patient environment and expand their professional careers by working as case managers. The case manager is removed from direct care delivery to coordinate overall patient services. This individual is also part of a multi-disciplinary team that continually assesses, evaluates and plans patient care. The assessment is based upon expectations regarding outcomes of care of the physician, nurse, and all other individuals involved in the care of the patient.

A multidisciplinary action plan (MAP) projects patient care outcomes for each day of hospitalization. Because the care plan is a group effort, it promotes greater satisfaction for the patient, family and health team members. These plans involve all patient care areas and specialities and cover a wide range of diagnoses or surgical procedures, such as neurosurgery, orthopedics, AIDS, general medicine, pediatrics, maternal/child health, oncology, detoxification, and rehabilitation. Ultimately, the model increases professional development and results in improved recruitment, motivation, and retention of staff (Ake et al, 1991).

Case managers, who are unit-based, coordinate the care being delivered by the registered nurses and nursing assistants working on the team. The manager also serves as a role model to the novice nurse or orientee. By consulting with less-experienced registered nurses, the manager helps improve the professionalism and clinical skills of the unit's personnel and promotes collegial relationships with all health care providers. Other responsibilities of the case manager include patient and family teaching and support and discharge planning with the social worker.

This model enhances the use of personnel by expanding support or ancillary staff role responsibilities. The nursing attendants who are included as part of the care team develop a better understanding of the medical and nursing needs of their patients.

The managed patient care model is an integral component of the organizational restructuring of patient care delivery. Because it is research-based and part of the planned change process, several clinical and quality care indicators are being evaluated to determine the effectiveness of this model. This model requires ongoing assessment of quality improvement data, job and patient satisfaction ratings, and length-of-stay data in order to adapt the practice principles and philosophy of the managed patient care model to the needs of the providers and recipients of acute health care services.

REFERENCES

Ake, J.M., Bower-Ferris, S., Cesta, T., Gould, D., Greenfield, J., Hayes, P., Maislin, G., and Mezey, M. (1991). The nursing initiatives program: Practice based models for care in hospitals. In *Differentiating Nursing Practice: Into the Twenty-First Century*. Kansas City, Mo.: American Academy of Nursing.

Cesta, T. (1991, November). *Managed Care,* personal correspondence and paper presented at the Annual Symposium on Health Services Research, New York.

Etheredge, M.L. (1989). *Collaborative Care Nursing Case Management.* Chicago: American Hospital Publishing, Inc. (American Hospital Association).

Zander, K. (1990). Managed care and nursing case management. In G.G. Mayer, M.J. Madden, & E. Lawrenz (Ed.), *Patient care delivery models* (pp. 37-61). Rockville, Md.: Aspen Publishers, Inc.

Zander, K. (1991, April). Presentation at *Nursing care management: Transcending walls opening gates,* Saint Joseph Medical Center, Wichita, Ks.

5

Within-the-Walls Case Management: A Nursing Hospital-Based Case Management Model

CHAPTER OVERVIEW

This chapter reviews various models of within-the-walls case management. This approach became popular when hospitals began restructuring to improve productivity, manage effective use of resources, lower costs, and maintain quality.

Preliminary findings show that this patient care delivery model can have a great effect on resource use and quality patient care. Daily assessment and evaluation of the patient's clinical care, reduced length of stay and other financial benefits, general applicability of this model, and improved nurse, physician, and patient satisfaction demonstrate the merit and relevancy of this approach to patient care delivery and professional practice.

COST-EFFECTIVE CARE

The changing nature of health care economics has forced hospitals to view case management as an alternative to the delivery of direct care services. Hospital-based case management is founded on traditional approaches. Its ensures the most appropriate use of services by patients. A case management system in the hospital setting avoids duplication and misuse of medical services, controls costs by reducing inefficient services, and improves the effectiveness of care delivery (Lavizzo-Mourey, 1987). Lavizzo-Mourey (1987), McIntosh (1987), and Henderson and Collard (1988) reported several advantages of hospital-based case management. First, the hospital setting offers a wide range of specialized skills that can be made available to both the provider and recipient of case management services. Second, because the majority of the resources needed for patient care are centralized within the acute care setting, early assessment of patient needs, planning and coordination of care delivery, and evaluation of alternative systems are enhanced. Third, because space and overhead costs are factored into hospital-based care, the management of expenditures associated with high-cost patients is minimized. Fourth, systems for monitoring and measuring the cost-effectiveness of case management arrangements are present within the hospital setting.

Many hospital-based case management systems have engaged registered nurses as case managers (Henderson & Collard, 1988; Henderson & Wallack, 1987; McIntosh, 1987). Nurse involvement in case management allows nurses to influence and direct the delivery and quality of patient care. Such involvement allows for more control, visibility, and recognition for nursing services delivered. The involvement also offers more consistent outcome attainment and demonstrates nursing personnel contributions to patient care (Zander, 1988a).

Because it would be virtually impossible to cover all patient models of nursing case management that may currently exist, this chapter will focus on some of the systems that have served as the foundation for the development of within-the-walls case management. The chapter will also highlight those approaches to patient care delivery and professional practice that have been published and have received national attention.

PRIMARY NURSE CASE MANAGEMENT MODEL

Nursing case management has emerged in the acute care setting as a professional model of practice. One model, characterized as a primary nurse case management model, has been used at the New England Medical Center in Boston, Massachusetts. Stetler (1987), Woldum (1987), and Zander (1988a, b, 1990), have identified the following factors that distinguish this case management system of care.

Primary nurse case management is based on the concept of managed care. Managed care is defined as care that is unit-based, outcome-oriented, dependent on a designated time frame, and focused on the appropriate use of resources for both the inpatient and outpatient population.

Primary nurse case management services and case loads are designated for specific patient case types or case mixes. Some examples of case types coordinated by primary nurse case management are cardiac, leukemia, pediatric gastrointestinal disorders, some gynecological, stroke, and craniotomy patients.

Nursing case managers are the primary care givers for patients. The managers provide direct care to patients in their case loads while the patients are housed in their units and continue to coordinate the care of these patients throughout hospitalization, regardless of the patient's physical location.

The process of care is monitored by the use of case management plans, which include DRG length of stay; critical path reports, which outline the components of appropriate care; and variance analysis, which ensures the continuous evaluation of patient care activities.

Care is coordinated through collaborative group practice arrangements across geographic units, case consultation, and health care team meetings. Patient discharge planning is outlined before admission and updated throughout hospitalization until the time of discharge.

The New England Medical Center's nursing case management model presents an innovative alternative to the delivery of nursing care within the acute care setting. The model has evolved since its introduction and has been widely adapted. The development of Care Maps increases the potential for evaluating the cost-effectiveness and quality of care standards proposed by this model. Care Maps have expanded on case management plans and critical paths by focusing on both standards of care and practice for a specific case type, responding to variances in the delivery of care, linking Continuous Quality Improvement (CQI) to practices, and integrating resource allocation, patient care outcomes, and cost reimbursement systems (Zander, 1991; Zander 1992a; Zander, 1992b).

The competence and experience of the case manager is critical to the effective delivery of patient care services (Henderson & Wallack, 1987). The Case Management Model at New England Medical Center, along with most nurse case management programs, primarily uses registered nurses as case managers. A case manager must have at least 1 year of nursing experience and charge responsibilities and must demonstrate leadership ability. Henderson and Wallack (1987) and Henderson and Collard (1988) recommend that to ensure cost-effective care and quality assurance standards, the nurse case manager should have expertise related to the care of designated types of patients and specific diagnostic categories. Because of the model's reliance on a primary nursing care delivery system, staffing mix allocation was not differentiated in the New England Medical Center's model. Some case management programs have successfully employed a variety of personnel other than professional nursing staff. Studies are needed that determine the best staffing mix for nursing case management programs. Contrary to what Zander (1990) reported about the nursing case management model at the New England Medical Center, a recent study in another institution has shown a preliminary increase in direct nursing care hours and greater use of resources during the initial phase of hospitalization. These changes resulted in an overall decrease in length of stay, an increase in patient turnover, and a potential increase in patient revenues generated for the hospital (Cohen, 1991).

LEVELED PRACTICE MODEL

Another nursing case management model, identified as the leveled practice model, has focused on the management and coordination of patient care needs. This system differs from the primary nurse case management model in that the case manager's functions are focused on the management activities of patient care and not on the responsibility for patient care delivery (Loveridge, Cummings & O'Malley, 1988; O'Malley & Cummings, 1988). A work group consisting of registered nurses, licensed practical nurses, and nurses' aides, provides direct care on a specific patient unit. The professional nurse is designated as the case manager and is responsible for coordinating and monitoring patient care of an assigned case load through collaboration with the work group, patient, family, and interdisciplinary health team members. In addition, the case manager relies on information related to case mix, hospital costs, patient resource use, insurance, and reimbursement data (O'Malley & Cummings, 1988).

The leveled case management model has promoted differentiated practice arrangements by delineating functional role responsibility and accountability between those nurses with baccalaureate degrees and those with associate degrees (Loveridge, Cummings & O'Malley, 1988). Differentiated competency levels in nursing practice were classified extensively by Primm (1986). Because of the principles inherent in leveled practice case management, the role of the professional staff nurse changes to an autonomous one. Consequently, this change in practice places different obligations on the nurse manager. The nurse manager's role becomes what MacGregor-Burns (1978) described as transformational leadership, which is focused on teaching, mentoring, and coaching activities. In the leveled practice nursing case management model, management responsibility emphasized overall administrative and fiscal support, as well as patient outcome assessment and quality care improvement (Loveridge, Cummings & O'Malley, 1988; O'Malley & Cummings, 1988).

PRIMARY CASE MANAGEMENT

The primary case management model, which was developed and implemented at Hermann Hospital in Houston, embraced the primary nursing philosophy of care and used a clinical career ladder for registered nurses (Cavouras, Walts, Taylor, Garner & Bordelon, 1990). The clinical ladder consisted of six levels of clinical expertise, which progressed from a patient-focused orientation at the beginning levels to interdisciplinary and general service practice responsibility and accountability as nurse case managers at the top level.

The primary case management model used unit-based case managers who were responsible for coordinating, developing, and evaluating the delivery and the quality of patient care. Staff nurses and nurse extenders were the ones who provided the care that was established on the basis of standard protocols. The care plans outlined the daily care requirements and activities and served as a mechanism to monitor and evaluate issues related to quality and patient care resource use for nursing and hospitalwide support services such as laboratory, pharmacy, and respiratory therapy. Quality improvement was monitored as well through unit-based quality assurance programs.

Cost effectiveness, quality of care, and nurses' job satisfaction were also evaluated through retrospective variance analysis of patient charges and length of hospital stay, quality-assurance monitoring, and nurse satisfaction surveys. To date, no data have been published.

SAINT JOSEPH MERCY HOSPITAL'S PONTIAC PROJECT AND MERCY HOSPITAL'S PORT HURON PROJECT

Both Saint Joseph Mercy Hospital and Mercy Hospital served as case management project demonstration sites and were part of the Mercy Health Services Consortium.

The Pontiac project a collaborative practice model was implemented using case management in the medical-surgical division (Wesley & Easterling, 1991). Critical paths and patient care teaching plans were used to focus care needs and resource use on high risk patients. These plans involved patient, family, and care team assessments. Variations in patient care were monitored to ensure continuity. A competency-based clinical advancement design was developed to maintain the high level of leadership, commitment, and expertise needed for the case manager role.

Preliminary evaluation of this model revealed increased collaboration and enhanced professional relationships among nurses and physicians. Additional benefits of this collaborative effort included more efficient and improved clinical programs, improved quality care, and greater professional respect and autonomy.

The Mercy Hospital Port Huron Project, which is still under development, will incorporate a case management approach into a community health care system (McClelland & Foster, 1991). This case management model will be used for oncology patients. In this system, health care delivery will operate on a continuum and will integrate service aspects related to hospitalization, home care, and hospice. Collaborative practice arrangements will be interdisciplinary to ensure continuous, quality patient care. Community education programs, home care, and respite services will also be provided. Monitoring systems will help evaluate job satisfaction, cost, and quality of patient care.

TUCSON MEDICAL CENTER CASE MANAGEMENT MODEL

A case management model was developed at Tucson Medical Center to address both the cost and quality aspects of patient care delivery (Del Togno-Armanasco, Olivas & Harter, 1989). This approach incorporated elements of the New England Medical Center's Case Management Model and differentiated practice models in addition to basic philosophic practice components of primary nursing and shared governance.

Called Collaborative Case Management, the primary focus of this model was on standardizing the use of patient care resources and the delivery of services during the patient's hospitalization for selected DRG case types. Both patient mix and service volume management strategies were used to attain cost-effective, quality patient care (Olivas, Del Togno-Armanasco, Erickson, & Harter, 1989a).

A Collaborative Case Management Plan (CCMP) and a MAP are used to identify the contributions of all health care providers and support a unit-specific standard of patient care. Variations from practice standards are also monitored and evaluated.

Hospitalwide and unit-specific multidisciplinary practice committees were established to assist in clinical decision-making and overall evaluation processes of the patient care model. These groups consisted of physical therapists, dietitians, social workers, physicians, and home care professionals (Olivas, Del Togno-Armanasco, Erickson & Harter, 1989b). Patients were encouraged to participate and were included in the planning of their care regimen, which was carried out on a continuous basis from the time of admission to after discharge.

Various evaluation mechanisms were developed to measure the potential impact of this case management model on outcomes of care. A patient-satisfaction questionnaire and a retrospective chart review have been implemented along with a physician-satisfaction-with-care questionnaire to ascertain variables related to patient care and job satisfaction. Information on cost of care, rate of absenteeism, and staff turnover was also collected. Findings showed increased satisfaction with both nursing and medical care (at the .05 alpha level) for case-managed, total-hip-replacement patients, coronary bypass, and valvular-surgery patients. There was no turnover among nurse case managers and a marked decrease in turnover rates was demonstrated for nursing staff on the oncology and orthopedic units.

Outcome data also showed a decreased length of stay among patients who underwent total-hip and knee replacements. The decrease was 3.48 and 2.82 days respectively over a 3½-year period. Length of stay for valvular replacement and coronary bypass patients also decreased. In addition, a positive cost variance of $9,273 was realized for the valvular replacement and coronary bypass patient populations (Del Togno-Armanasco, 1992).

SAINT MICHAEL HOSPITAL'S COORDINATED CARE MODEL

Coordinated care is another innovative case management approach that was implemented at Saint Michael Hospital in Milwaukee, Wisconsin. With the use of critical paths and a comprehensive variance analysis system, this model expanded upon the practice concepts of nursing case management from the New England Medical Center's model (Sinnen & Schifalacqua, 1991).

The coordinated care approach demonstrated organizational effectiveness through a decrease in costs related to shorter length of stay and a reduction in hospital-associated charges (Sinnen & Schifalacqua, 1991). An additional gain included increased communication across all disciplines involved in patient care delivery.

Within the last 3 years a change was instituted from the modified primary nursing delivery system to the dyad model. The dyad care delivery modification involved a partnership between a registered nurse and technical assistant who cared for a specific number of patients (see Chapter 2 for description). In addition, Saint Michael's within-the wall model is in the fourth generation of multidisciplinary critical paths. The patient action plan is a permanent part of the medical record and includes patient outcomes, multidisciplinary interventions, teaching record, and nursing care plan (M. Schifalacqua, 1992).

REFERENCES

Cavouras, C.A., Walts, L., Taylor, S., Garner, A., & Bordelon, P. (1990). Alternative Delivery System: Primary case management. In G. Mayer, M. Madden, & E. Lawrenz (Ed.), *Patient Care Delivery Models* (pp. 275-282), Rockville, Md. Aspen Publishers, Inc.

Cohen, E. (1991). Nursing case management: Does it pay? *Journal of Nursing Administration, 21*(4), 20-25.

Del Togno-Armanasco, V., Olivas, G., & Harter, S. (1989). Developing an integrated nursing case management model. *Nursing Management, 20*(5), 26-29.

Del Togno-Armanasco, V. (1992). [Collaborative Case Management: Outcome data]. Unpublished raw data.

Henderson, M.G., & Collard, A. (1988). Measuring quality in medical case management programs. *Quality Review Bulletin, 14*(2), 33-39.

Henderson, M.G., & Wallack, S.S. (1987). Evaluating case management for catastrophic illness. *Business and Health, 4*(3), 741.

Lavizzo-Mourey, R. (1987). Hospital based case management. *DRG Monitor, 5*(1), 1-8.

Loveridge, C., Cummings, S., & O'Malley, J. (1988). Developing case management in a primary nursing system. *Journal of Nursing Administration, 18*(10), 36-39.

MacGregor-Burns, J. (1978). *Leadership.* New York: Harper & Row.

McClelland, M., & Foster, D. (1991). The Mercy Hospital, Port Huron Project. *Nursing Administration Quarterly, 15*(4), 58-60.

McIntosh, L. (1987). Hospital based case management. *Nursing Economics, 5*(5), 232-236.

Olivas, G., Del Togno-Armanasco, V., Erickson, J.R., & Harter, S. (1989a). Case management: A bottom-line care delivery model: Part I: The concept. *Journal of Nursing Administration, 19*(11), 16-20.

Olivas, G., Del Togno-Armanasco, V., Erickson, J.R., & Harter, S. (1989b). Case management: A bottom-line care delivery model: Part II: Adaptation of the model. *Journal of Nursing Administration, 19*(12), 12-17.

O'Malley, J., & Cummings, S. (1988). Nursing case management, part III: Implementing case management. *Aspen's Advisor for Nurse Executives, 3*(7), 8-9.

Primm, P.L. (1986). Entry into practice: Competency statements for BSNs and ADNs. *Nursing Outlook, 34*(3), 135-137.

Schifalacqua, M. (1992). Personal communication.

Sinnen, M.T., & Schifalacqua, M. (1991). Coordinated care in a community hospital. *Nursing Management, 22*(3), 38-42.

Stetler, C.B. (1987). The case manager's role: A preliminary evaluation. *Definition, 2*(3), 1-4.

Wesley, M.L., & Easterling, A. (1991). The St. Joseph Mercy Hospital, Pontiac Project. *Nursing Administration Quarterly, 15*(4), 50-54.

Woldum, K. (1987). Critical paths: Marking the course. *Definition, 2*(3), 1-4.

Zander, K. (1988a). Managed care within acute care settings: Design and implementation via nursing case management. *Health Care Supervisor, 6*(2), 24-43.

Zander, K. (1988b). Nursing care management: Strategic management of cost and quality outcomes. *Journal of Nursing Administration, 18*(5), 23-30.

Zander, K. (1990). Managed care and nursing case management. In G.G. Mayer, M.J. Madden, & E. Lawrenz (Ed.), *Patient care delivery models* (pp. 37-61). Rockville, Md. Aspen Publishers, Inc.

Zander, K. (1991, Fall). Care Maps TM: The core of cost/quality care. *The New Definition, 6*(3), 1-3.

Zander, K. (1992a, Winter). Physicians, Care Maps and collaboration. *The New Definition, 7*(1), 1-4.

Zander, K. (1992b, Spring). Quantifying, managing, and improving quality, Part I: How Care Maps link CQI to the patient. *The New Definition, 1*(2), 1-3.

Beyond-the-Walls Case Management

CHAPTER OVERVIEW

Nursing case management approaches have grown in sophistication and diversity as evidenced by their emergence in community-based programs and capitated system arrangements. A beyond-the-walls program offers magnificent opportunities for professional nursing to control and manage health care resources and quality of patient care. Such a program also provides multiple advantages for the coordination and integration of outcomes and costs. The nursing profession's increased emphasis on the patient strengthens its power base and reconfirms its professional commitment to society.

Beyond-the-walls case management represents yet another example of the versatility and applicability of the case management model. This community-based approach has shown great promise in reshaping nursing practice and health care management. Examples of some of the more prominent models are presented in the next section.

CARONDELET SAINT MARY'S NURSING HEALTH MAINTENANCE ORGANIZATION

One of the most integrated and cost-effective systems of nursing case management was developed at Carondelet Saint Mary's Hospital and Health Center in Tucson, Arizona. It is one of the first nursing case management models to relate its practice to nursing theory. The theoretic constructs of Newman's Health as Expanding Consciousness model is used to help guide the nurse case manager in the delivery of patient care and support services (Newman, Lamb & Michaels, 1991).*

This model evolved from a decentralized home care program and nursing network system that provided a multitude of services in a variety of settings

---

*The theoretic constructs of other nursing theorists such as Orem and Rogers are also applicable to case management models.

(Ethridge, 1987; Ethridge, 1991; Ethridge & Lamb, 1989). The services administered in the original system included acute or inpatient care, long-term extended care, home health care, hospice, rehabilitation, primary preventive, and ambulatory care (Ethridge, 1991; Ethridge & Lamb, 1989).

Also referred to as home-based case management, this former system reduced the fragmentation associated with preadmission assessment, discharge planning, post-discharge follow-up, and hospital readmission (Health Care Advisory Board, 1990). Based on managed care concepts, this system gave a professional nurse case manager (PNCM) responsibility for coordinating, planning, and evaluating patient care and necessary resources. This case manager was also a member of a professional group practice. The responsibilities of the case manager included:

Identifying those patients in the hospital setting that are at risk for readmission, such as the elderly, patients who are chronically ill, and those who have limited social or financial support.

Coordinating patient education related to self-care.

Coordinating community and agency resources through multidisciplinary relationships.

Making home visits to assess, monitor, and evaluate care.

Providing emotional support, counseling, and necessary referrals.

Serving as a liaison and patient advocate to the physicians, nurses, and community in the event of rehospitalization (Health Care Advisory Board, 1990).

Cost data showed reductions in length of stay for both acutely and chronically ill patients. The most significant outcome was that the assessment, coordination, planning, and monitoring associated with professional nursing case management led to the appropriate use of medical intervention technology, timely readmissions to the hospital, reduced inpatient severity levels, subsequent decreases in length of stay, and increased accessibility to alternative health care delivery options. These factors helped prevent unnecessary hospitalization (Ethridge, 1991; Ethridge & Lamb, 1989; Health Care Advisory Board, 1990).

Building upon the success of the first approach, a nursing HMO was established to provide health care and support services to the elderly, chronically ill, and disabled individuals within a Medicare Senior Plan Contract (Ethridge, 1991; Michaels, 1991; Michaels, 1992). Enrollees in this health plan receive the many services provided by PNCMs who are also part of a multidisciplinary health care team. Services include initial admission screening to the hospital, consultations and referrals, continuous monitoring of patient care needs, health assessments, and health education. Various services are also provided through dedicated Nursing Community Health Centers that are run by nurse practitioners and offer a range of health promotion and educational services (Ethridge, 1991; Michaels, 1992).

Client information as well as cost and quality data are collected and analyzed through a computerized information system. This system establishes a mechanism for tracking service use in various settings (Lamb, 1992b). Preliminary studies have demonstrated a decrease in the costs of hospitalization, reduction in patient length of stay, and cost savings related to early nursing assessment, intervention, and managed care for high-risk patients (Lamb, 1992a). Both quantitative and qualitative variables are being analyzed on an ongoing basis (Lamb, 1992a). These include analyzing patterns related to hospital use, monitoring frequency and use of case management services, and explicating the experiences of the clients as they go through the care process (Ethridge, 1991; Michaels, 1991; Michaels, 1992; Newman, Lamb & Michaels, 1991). In addition, a system is being developed to identify the complete cost of nursing case management. This will be a crucial element for ensuring greater reimbursement in the future (Lamb, 1992b).

Although the original emphasis of the Saint Mary's program was on service delivery, a more focused approach has been implemented toward evaluation and research (Lamb, 1992b). This is reflective of what Lamb (1992a) states as "an awareness of the major conceptual and methodological issues facing those who practice and attempt to study nurse case management" (see also Chapter 16). Process and outcome measurements related to cost effectiveness, quality of care, and customer satisfaction are currently under investigation (Lamb, 1992a).

Lamb (1992a) identifies five factors for guiding future research in nursing case management. These factors include:

Linking studies on cost effectiveness and efficiency to the quality of patient care delivery.

Extending the research focus to include outcomes that encompass an entire spectrum of care and services in all settings.

Generalizing research findings to broader interest groups and concerns to meet long-range social, economic, and health care needs.

Encouraging and facilitating diverse research methodology.

Focusing on the process elements of research to enhance nursing case management care.

SAINT JOSEPH MEDICAL CENTER'S COMMUNITY-BASED NURSING CASE MANAGEMENT

A community-based nursing case management system was implemented at Saint Joseph Medical Center in Wichita, Kansas. This system was modeled after the system at Carondelet Saint Mary's and maintains a multidisciplinary, multiservice responsibility for the coordination of services and management of the patient. The system originally included only the high at risk, the frail elderly, and/or the chronically ill (Rogers, Riordan & Swindle, 1991). "[The system] is now addressing several other patient populations including psychiatric, high-risk pregnancy and neonates, as well as chronically ill younger adults and children. Staff have also done considerable work on collaboration with local schools of nursing on educational issues and on the incorporation of other disciplines into the model. These include social work, respiratory care, dieticians, and a protocol for hospital chaplaincy students who also do rotations with them" (Rogers, 1992).

Outcome variables related to the number of hospital readmissions, length of stay, reimbursement or payment arrangements, and referral relationships are analyzed through a fully automated data base. Preliminary results demonstrate cost savings related to reduction in hospital admissions and length of stay. Future projects that integrate nursing diagnosis and standards of care will be designed to create a national nursing data base retrieval system that would enhance the documentation and analysis of this model (Rogers, Riordan & Swindle, 1991).

REFERENCES

Ethridge, P. (1987). Building successful nursing care delivery systems for the future. In National Commission on Nursing Implementation Project (Ed.), *Post-Conference Papers Second Invitational Conference* (pp. 91-99). Milwaukee: W.K. Kellogg Foundation.

Ethridge, P., & Lamb, G. (1989). Professional nursing case management improves quality, access and costs. *Nursing Management, 20*(3), 30-35.

Ethridge, P. (1991). A nursing HMO: Carondelet St. Mary's experience. *Nursing Management, 22*(7), 22-27.

Health Care Advisory Board (1990). Tactic #6 "Home-Based" case management. *Superlative Clinical Quality: Special Review of Pathbreaking Ideas, Clinical Quality (Volume I)* (pp. 71-94) Washington, D.C.: The Advisory Board Company.

Lamb, G. (1992a). Conceptual and methodological issues in nurse case management research. *Advances in Nursing Science, 15*(2), 16-24.

Lamb, G. (1992b). Personal communication.

Michaels, C. (1991). A nursing HMO—10 months with Carondelet St. Mary's Hospital-based nurse case management. *Aspen's Advisor for Nurse Executives, 6*(11), 1-4.

Michaels, C. (1992). Carondelet St. Mary's nursing enterprise. *Nursing Clinics of North America, 27*(1), 77-85.

Newman, M., Lamb, G., & Michaels, C. (1991). Nurse case management. The coming together of theory and practice. *Nursing and Health Care, 12*(8), 404-408.

Rogers, M., Riordan, J., & Swindle, D. (1991). Community-based nursing case management pays off. *Nursing Management, 22*(3), 30-34.

Rogers, M. (1992). Personal communication.

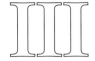

COST-EFFECTIVENESS OF CASE MANAGEMENT AND MAINTAINING CONTROL: SOCIOECONOMIC AND POLITICAL IMPLICATIONS

Patient Demographics Affecting Health Care

CHAPTER OVERVIEW

Recent shifts in the nation's demographics are causing substantial changes in the delivery of health care. Both the increasing elderly population and the AIDS epidemic have prompted health care workers to look for alternatives to the traditional approaches of acute patient care and have fostered the growth of integrative models such as case management. The increasing prevalence of chronic illness and disability associated with the demographic changes are also influencing public health policy as we shift our resources from acute to chronic care.

Recently enacted legislation has provided for the civil rights and liberties of those individuals with chronic illness and has supported much needed community-based and long-term health care delivery systems. Many businesses and corporations have begun to develop programs and services that will help them adapt to the long-range social, economic, and health care implications of the growing number of elderly or those with Acquired Immune Deficiency Syndrome (AIDS).

AGING PATIENT POPULATION

The Department of Health and Human Services (1990) predicts that by the year 2020, 7 million Americans will be older than 85 years of age. In the 1990s the percentage of men and women who are 80 years old is expected to increase 30% to 45% for men and 24% to 36% for women (Dimond, 1989; Exter, 1990). This increase in number and percentage of older individuals is primarily due to advances in research, technology, and preventive treatments that have resulted in marked declines in mortality rates associated with cancer, cardiovascular disease, diabetes, stroke, and hypertension (National Center for Health Statistics, 1985; Olshansky, 1985).

Rogers, Rogers, and Belanger (1989) found a correlation between dependency and age. Their study indicates that an increase in age results in a corresponding rise in functional dependency related to basic activities of daily living. Further-

49

more, once dependency sets in, the likelihood of returning to an independent status decreases. An example of this is that although females have a longer life expectancy than males, the study shows that much of that time is spent in dependent situations, which increases the morbidity of this population group (Manton, 1988; Schneider & Brody, 1983).

Statistical projections show that by the year 2044, 7.3 million people will have dependent lifestyles (Rogers, Rogers & Belanger, 1989). Another projection indicates that by the year 2040, the elderly population will account for 45% of health care expenditures (Callahan, 1987).

With advanced age, there is also a proportionate growth in the incidence of chronic and degenerative illnesses. These factors, along with increased dependency and disability, intensify the need and demand for increased utilization of health care services (Goldsmith, 1989; Guralnik, Yanagishita & Schneider, 1988).

As highlighted by the National Center for Health Statistics (1987), 1.3 million of those older than 65 live in nursing homes. Of those, 46% are older than 85 years of age. By the year 2040, it is estimated that 2.8 million people, age 85 and older, will require institutional care (Guralnik et al., 1988). These data indicate that the aging population will have a significant effect on long-term and skilled nursing care.

Increased longevity and its concomitant effects have encouraged new approaches to the delivery of health care services. Nursing case management, managed care programs, and community-based home care are some examples of alternative approaches to meeting the health care needs of the elderly. These approaches lend themselves to scrutiny and analysis related to cost-effectiveness and the value and quality of services delivered.

In an extensive review of home- and community-based long-term care programs, Weissert, Cready, and Pawelak (1988) found that there were greater total expenditures and no statistically significant cost savings related to home- and community-based care. In fact, an analysis of the effectiveness of various programs showed that even though there were reductions in admissions to institutional care settings, these findings were significant for only a small group of patients who had an obvious need for home-based care. This group consisted of the disabled, chronically ill, and frail elderly.

The study showed, however, that within this patient population, preadmission assessment and screening of those individuals at risk for institutionalization effectively reduced nursing home use. This finding was supported in studies that evaluated the effectiveness of community-based programs in preventing hospitalization. Again, it was shown that more specific identification and evaluation of patient requirements of care decreased the need for and length of inpatient treatment and hospitalization.

One major benefit of community- and home-based care was found in its beneficial and significant effect on the psychosocial well-being and satisfaction of patients and care providers. The community- or home-based care proved better at meeting the patients' needs for physical and social activities as well as medical, mental health, and educational requirements (Weissert, 1985).

Another study, conducted by Roos, Shapiro, and Tate (1989), indicated that only 5% of the elderly are extensive users of health care in both the inpatient, acute care, and nursing home settings. The expenditures associated with this care are higher during the individual's last year of life. However, 45% of the elderly population makes large demands on the health care system, and these demands result in greater expenditures.

One recommendation for decreasing the chance of hospitalization is to provide the elderly with a geriatric specialist. Early assessment and evaluation by such a specialist might help reduce the incidence of hospitalization, which in turn decreases costs. In addition, continuous monitoring of discharged patients through home care, community-based care, long-term care, and primary preventive services can be cost-effective and aid in the transition to a more independent life status.

It is clear that to plan effectively for future health care needs of the elderly and disabled population, changes in the delivery of health care services and benefits are needed. Resources are now being shifted from acute care and long-term institutional care to home care, community-based services, respite centers, nurse-run HMOs and care centers, case management, and rehabilitation programs (Dimond, 1989; Hollinger & Brugler, 1991; Maraldo & Solomon, 1987).

To maintain control of some of the long-range, economic and social implications, major business groups and corporations are beginning to develop and offer resource and referral services to employees who have caretaking responsibilities for elderly and dependent family members (Buchsbaum, 1991; Peterson, 1992). Called eldercare, these programs provide a range of services including counseling, family leave plans, position reinstatement, flexible work schedules, automated office arrangements that make it possible for employees to work at home, subsidized health care benefits, and reimbursement for adult day-care.

Benefits of such an approach include decreased work-related conflicts; lowered costs associated with recruitment, training, and absenteeism of personnel; and increased productivity, loyalty, and commitment to the organization. Referral services have also helped decrease the costs of health services associated with deferred spending, out-of-pocket expenses, lost time, and stress (Buchsbaum, 1991; Peterson, 1992).

HIV INFECTION

Statistics from the U.S. Centers for Disease Control show that 1.5 to 2 million Americans are infected with HIV and more than 30% of those people will develop AIDS by 1993 (Mason, 1990; U.S. Center for Disease Control, 1989). It is estimated that there will be a fourfold increase in HIV and HIV-related infections in the next four to five years (Mason, 1990).

There is substantial evidence that the rapid spread of HIV will result in increased hospitalizations and greater use of more complex health care resources. Medicaid alone is projected to spend 47 billion dollars on individuals with HIV (Scitovsky, 1988).

Several studies indicate that the United States will spend about $10 billion in direct cost (i.e., hospitalization, home and hospice care) for the treatment of AIDS in 1991 (American Hospital Association, 1986; Lyon, 1988; Scitovsky & Rice, 1987). This estimate includes the cost of hospitalization, home health care, hospice, and outpatient care as well as costs related to disability and chronicity.

The initial length of hospitalization averages 30 to 60 days, with cumulative acute-care treatment lasting up to 170 days (Hardy, Rauch, Echenberg, et al, 1986; Sedaka & O'Reilly, 1986). On average, a person with AIDS is hospitalized three to four times. These hospitalizations occur in the early and late stages of illness (Scitovsky, Cline & Lee, 1986).

Because AIDS is chronic, debilitating, and terminal, it places a substantial burden on the health care system (Benjamin, 1988). Home care, community-based services, hospice, and case management provide alternatives to hospitalization. The availability and applicability of these resources are being considered in the formulation of public policy regarding the delivery of health care services for individuals with AIDS (Fox, 1989).

Various strategies are under consideration to improve accessibility of AIDS care settings. Hospitals have created designated AIDS units where registered nurses coordinate, plan, and evaluate the delivery of care (Chow, 1989; Fox, Aiken & Messikomer, 1990). Some institutions, such as the San Francisco General Hospital, have implemented comprehensive care programs through multidisciplinary, collaborative efforts with outpatient and community-based services, and home care agencies (Volberding, 1985). These initiatives, along with the improvement in the treatment and management protocols, have worked toward decreasing the length of stay for AIDS patients, thereby affecting the overall care and cost-effectiveness of this group (Fox, 1986).

The effectiveness of ambulatory and community-based programs for AIDS care is being evaluated in many federal, state, and private foundation-sponsored projects (Benjamin, 1988; Fox, 1986). The programs could mean cost savings by reducing the need for inpatient hospital care resources and services.

Hospice care is another promising alternative for AIDS treatment. Using a multidisciplinary team approach, the hospice setting provides for the psychosocial needs of both the patient and caregiver (Benjamin, 1988). The emphasis of hospice care is on reducing time spent in institutional care and eliminating the need for acute medical intervention.

Studies done by Mor and Kidder (1985) on the cost-effectiveness of hospice care show savings related to decreases in inpatient length of stay and use of hospital resources. Such decreases are possibly due to the shift in caregiving responsibility to the patient's community, family, and significant others.

Case management presents an additional option for planning nonacute care services and interventions for individuals with AIDS. Capitman, Haskins, & Bernstein (1986), and Spitz (1987), demonstrated the effectiveness and efficiency of a well-integrated case management system. Their studies show that through comprehensive targeting and planning and integration of inpatient, ambulatory, and community-based services, the medical and social needs of AIDS patients can be met. Case management also provides flexibility in service options and reduces the inappropriateness, overuse, and inefficiency associated with hospital and medical care of the chronically ill (Schramm, 1990). Other hospital-based nursing case management models dedicated to AIDS care have also been effective in delivering less-expensive quality care (American Nurses Association, 1988).

Since AIDS presents enormous acute and long-term care needs, business firms have begun to develop and provide employee education and assistance programs, counseling services, nondiscriminatory employment policies, and flexible work schedules. Corporations have also begun to comply with federal, state, and local infection control guidelines (McDonald, 1990; Mello, 1991).

The passage of the Americans With Disabilities Act (ADA) in 1992 will also help to ensure the rights of HIV- and AIDS-infected people in the workplace. The benefits and entitlements under this act include opportunities for employment, access to public services, accessible transportation, and a mechanism of communication with employers to support non-discriminatory policies, confidentiality, and ongoing education (Feldblum, 1991; LaPlante, 1991).

REFERENCES

American Hospital Association (1986). *Infection Control and Environmental Safety Committee. AIDS.* Chicago: American Hospital Association.

American Nurses Association (1988). *Nursing case management.* Kansas City, Mo.: American Nurses Association.

Benjamin, A.E. (1988). Long-term care and AIDS: Perspectives from experience with the elderly. *The Milbank Quarterly, 66*(3), 415-443.

Buchsbaum, S. (1991). Sending "care" packages to the workplace. *Business and Health, 9*(5), 56-69.

Callahan, D. (1987). *Setting limits: Medical goals in an aging society.* New York: Simon and Schuster.

Capitman, J.A., Haskins, B., & Bernstein, J. (1986). Case management approaches in community oriented long-term care demonstrations. *Gerontologist, 26,* 398-404.

Chow, M. (1989). Nursing's response to the challenge of AIDS. *Nursing Outlook, 37*(2), 82-83.

Department of Health and Human Services. (1990). *Healthy People 2000.* Washington, D.C.: DHHS.

Dimond, M. (1989). Health care and the aging population. *Nursing Outlook, 37*(2), 76-77.

Exter, T. (1990, June). How big will the older market be? *American Demographics,* 30-36.

Feldblum, C. (1991). Employment Protections. *The Milbank Quarterly, 69*(Suppl. 1/2), 81-110.

Fox, D. (1986). AIDS and the American health policy: History and prospects of a crises of authority. *The Milbank Quarterly, 64,* 7-33.

Fox, D. (1989). Policy and epidemiology: Financing health services for the chronically ill and disabled, 1930-1990. *The Milbank Quarterly, 67*(Suppl. 2, Part 2), 257-287.

Fox, R., Aiken, L., & Messikomer, C. (1990). The culture of caring: AIDS and the nursing profession. *The Milbank Quarterly, 68*(Suppl. 2), 226-256.

Goldsmith, J. (1989). Radical prescription for hospitals. *Harvard Business Review, 89*(3), 104-111.

Guralnik, J., Yanagishita, M., & Schneider, E. (1988). Projecting the older population of the United States: Lessons from the past and prospects for the future. *The Milbank Quarterly, 66*(2), 283-308.

Hardy, A., Rauch, K., Echenberg, D., Morgan, W., & Curran, J.W. (1986). The economic impact of the first 10,000 cases of acquired immunodeficiency syndrome in the United States. *Journal of the American Medical Association, 225,* 209-211.

Hollinger, W., & Brugler, K. (1991). Managing resource use. *Healthcare Forum, 34*(6), 45-47.

LaPlante, M. (1991). The demographics of disability. *The Milbank Quarterly, 69*(Suppl. 1/2), 55-77.

Lyon, J. (1988). AIDS: What are the costs? Who will pay? *Nursing Economics, 6*(5), 241-244, 274.

Manton, K.G. (1988). A longitudinal study of functional change and mortality in the United States. *Journal of Gerontology, 43*(5), 153-161.

Maraldo, P., & Solomon, S. (1987). Nursing's window of opportunity. *Image, 19*(2), 83-86.

Mason, J. (1990). Current and future impact of HIV on the nation. In T.P. Phillips and D. Bloch (Eds.). *Nursing and the HIV epidemic: A national agenda. Proceedings of an Invitational Workshop,* October 1-3, 1989, (pp. 21-19). Washington, D.C.: U.S. Department of Health and Human Services.

McDonald, M. (1990). How to deal with AIDS in the workplace. *Business and Health, 8*(7), 12-22.

Mello, J. (1991, September). Getting to know about AIDS. *Business and Health, 9*(9), 88-89.

Mor, V., & Kidder, D. (1985). Cost savings in hospice: Final results of the National Hospice Study. *Health Services Research, 20,* 407-421.

National Center for Health Statistics. (1985). *Vital Statistics of the United States, 1980.* 2(pt. A., mortality). DHHS pub. no. (PHS) 85-1101. Washington, D.C.

National Center for Health Statistics. (1987). Use of nursing homes by the elderly, preliminary data from the 1985 National Nursing Home Survey, by E. Hing. *Vital and Health Statistics,* no. 135. DHHS pub. no. (PHS) 87-1250. Washington, D.C.

Olshansky, S.J. (1985). Pursuing longevity: Delay vs. elimination of degenerative diseases. *American Journal of Public Health, 75,* 754-757.

Peterson, H. (1992, February). Eldercare: More than company kindness. *Business & Health, 10*(2), 54-57.

Rogers, R., Rogers, A., & Belanger, A. (1989). Active life among the elderly in the United States: Multistate Life-table estimates and population projections. *The Milbank Quarterly, 67*(3-4), 370-411.

Roos, N., Shapiro, E., & Tate, R. (1989). Does a small minority of elderly account for a majority of healthcare expenditures? A sixteen-year perspective. *The Milbank Quarterly, 67*(3-4), 347-369.

Schneider, E., & Brody, J. (1983). Aging, natural death, and the compression of morbidity: Another view. *New England Journal of Medicine, 309*(14), 854-855.

Schramm, C. (1990). Health care industry problems call for cooperative solutions. *Healthcare Financial Management,* 54-61.

Scitovsky, A.A., Cline, M., & Lee, P.R. (1986). Medical care costs of patients with AIDS in San Francisco. *Journal of the American Medical Association, 256,* 3103-3106.

Scitovsky, A.A., & Rice, D. (1987). Estimates of the direct and indirect costs of acquired immuno-deficiency syndrome in the United States, 1985, 1986, and 1991. *Public Health Reports, 102*(1), 5-17.

Scitovsky, A.A. (1988). The economic impact of AIDS in the United States. *Health Affairs, 7*(4), 32-45.

Sedaka, S., & O'Reilly, M. (1986). The financial implications of AIDS. *Caring, 5*(6), 38-44.

Spitz, B. (1987). National survey of medicaid case management. *Health Affairs, 6,* 61-70.

U.S. Centers for Disease Control (1989, May 12). AIDS and human immunodeficiency virus infection in the United States: 1988 update. *Morbidity and Mortality Weekly Report, 38*(Suppl. 4), 1-6.

Volberding, P.A. (1985). The clinical spectrum of the acquired immunodeficiency syndrome: Implications for comprehensive patient care. *Annals of Internal Medicine, 103,* 729-732.

Weissert, W.G. (1985). Seven reasons why it is so difficult to make community-based long term care cost effective. *Health Services Research, 20*(4), 423-433.

Weissert, W.G., Cready, C., & Pawelak, J. (1988). The past and future of home- and community-based long term care. *The Milbank Quarterly, 66*(2), 309-388.

The Business of Health Care and the Prospective Payment System

CHAPTER OVERVIEW

Changes in consumer behavior, along with various government and private industry strategies, have started to change the health care delivery environment. Programs are being developed to increase access to care and to evaluate and monitor cost-effective outcomes. National health reform initiatives address universal access to care by working for changes in insurance coverage and benefits, reimbursement regulation, and alternative care arrangements. Quality and cost are also addressed through managed care and capitated payment approaches. Long-term care services are being sponsored both publicly and privately.

Collaboration among health care providers for policy formation and implementation, public and private support for health care planning and outcome research, and further development of alternative care delivery and clinical resource models are among the crucial factors needed to develop an accessible, effective, and socially responsive health care system.

COST CONTAINMENT

The incentives promoted by the prospective payment system not only affect the efficiency, safety, and quality of health care in the inpatient setting but also have a direct relationship to the cost containment efforts present in managed care arrangements (Jones, 1989; Sloan, Morrisey & Valvona, 1988). Increased enrollment in HMOs and other prepaid, coordinated health care plans, restructuring of the physician fee and payment schedule to provide incentives for the delivery of primary care services, the national drive for health care reform, and competition among alternative delivery systems to improve cost-effectiveness and quality lend to the influence of prospective payment initiatives.*

Prospective payment has also promoted a more efficient use of health care

---

*Enthoven & Kronick, 1989a; Enthoven & Kronick, 1989b; Ginsburg & Hackbarth, 1986; Swoap, 1984; Waldo, Levit & Lazenby, 1986; Wilensky, 1991.

resources and encouraged the study of outcomes to evaluate accessibility, management, and economic effectiveness of care (Jones, 1989; Sloan, Morrisey, & Valvona, 1988).

The economic effect of rising health care costs has taken its toll on the private sector through increases in group health insurance premium rates and changes in the structure of employee health care benefits. Mullen (1988) and Traska (1989) reported that employers are experiencing rate increases of 15% to 29% in their efforts to cover health care costs. According to the Hewitt Associates' survey, the double-digit inflation is due to an estimated 21.5% increase by insurance carriers in medical benefit costs (Hewitt Associates, 1989). Increases in premiums are driven primarily by rises in the cost, volume, and variations in health services and are fostered by medical technologic change, an inadequate reimbursement system, demographic changes of an aging population, AIDS, and chronic illness (Kramon, 1989; Welling, 1990).

The issue of escalating health care costs has entered both the political and economic arenas and has prompted furious debates in the public and private sectors over the provision of basic health care services (Hospitals, 1992). Advocates for a national health care policy have locked horns with those who support the rationing of health services. Attempts have been made by Congress to institute a national health insurance plan to ensure equal access to care (Altman & Rodmin, 1988; Reinhardt, 1987a; Reinhardt, 1987b). Legislative mandates and congressional bills that would provide health care coverage have been introduced as a means of rationing care through regulation and achieving control over government expenditures. State-mandated benefit laws offer a broad range of service coverage and access to mental health and substance abuse care, prenatal care, mammography, cancer screening, and major organ transplants.*

Many special interest groups have joined forces to propose reform in the current health care system. One such group, the American Medical Association, supports an employer-based health care plan, and another group from organized nursing, has endorsed a proposal titled *Nursing's Agenda for Health Care Reform*. The latter plan supports a consumer partnership with the health care provider regarding decisions about care; access to primary health care services via community-based settings; allocation of more resources to chronic and long-term care; increased access to nonphysician providers, such as nurse practitioners; wellness and prevention classes, public and private sector review and financing of health care; and managed care and case management arrangements (National League for Nursing, 1991).

Changes in payment structure have taken place in almost every sector of the health care industry. Many different strategies aimed at cost containment have been adopted by private corporations and insurance providers. Various efforts have focused on the redesigning of health insurance plans and policies, shifting the direct financial burden of health care expenditures to the federal government

---

*Brown, 1988; Davis, 1985; Dwyer, 1991; Eckholm, 1991; Frieden, 1991; Tallon, 1991; Thorpe, 1991; Traska, 1989.

and individual payer. This approach includes the following: a single-payer plan, which is a government-financed plan that insures all individuals; introduction of copayments and deductibles applied to health care services; cost sharing, in which employees share the costs of health care by paying for the care of convalescing patients and/or hospice care for the terminally ill; catastrophic health plans, which provide coverage for high cost illnesses; second opinions for surgical interventions; and primary prevention and stress management programs aimed at controlling smoking, alcohol use, and hypertension.*

As an effective strategy for controlling health care costs, major corporations have also encouraged participation in comprehensive, capitated rate plans, such as HMOs, and PPOs. In these managed care plans, providers set an amount to cover all of their enrollees' health care needs. A percentage of that payment is put into a risk pool to ensure against unexpected expenditures. Providers assume a certain element of risk in exchange for the opportunity to benefit from lower costs, an integrated care system, and management savings (Brown, 1988; Christensen, 1991; Hicks, Stallmeyer & Coleman, 1992; O'Connor, 1991).

Another initiative, called *managed competition,* finances health insurance coverage through large businesses. The employer is required to purchase insurance or pay a payroll tax for a public (government) sponsor. This system promotes competition among private insurers and ensures quality improvement standards (Enthoven & Kronick, 1989a; Enthoven & Kronick, 1989b; Garland, 1991). All these health care delivery arrangements focus on both primary and secondary prevention, thereby increasing positive health outcomes and reducing costs (Hospitals, 1988; Luft, 1978; Luft, 1982; Rosenberg et al, 1991; Sloss, et al, 1987).

Another response to the problems of financing health care benefits is assuring the employer's involvement in managing the delivery of health care services. Providers are developing and participating in corporate health care programs that monitor cost and use of health care services. Those services that are monitored include preadmission testing, which has been shown to reduce inpatient stays, utilization review, monitoring of catastrophic illness and injury through medical case management programs, and mandatory employer-sponsored health insurance that would extend both private and public insurance coverage through various financial arrangements.† Such monitoring programs have helped reduce and eliminate medical inefficiency and have improved the effectiveness of care delivery.

Businesses have also begun to form health care coalitions that purchase health care services and offer them at a discount to their members. These coalitions guarantee accessible health care services, cost-effective delivery, and quality care. Some of the services provided by the coalitions include workers' compensation, inpatient and outpatient programs, primary prevention and treatment, and case management services (Bell, 1991).

---

*Brown, 1988; Frieden, 1991; Gilman & Bucco, 1987; Herzlinger & Schwartz, 1985; Herzlinger & Calkins, 1986; Peres, 1992.

†Aaron, 1991; Brown, 1988; Dalton, 1987; Dentzer, 1991; Herzlinger & Schwartz, 1985; Herzlinger, 1985; Herzlinger & Calkins, 1986; Peres, 1992.

NON-NURSING CASE MANAGEMENT MODELS

The primary focus of the case management model is to improve patient outcomes and control costs through the organization and coordination of health care services. The underlying economic premises of case management are dependent on the linkage to case management strategies developed by the private sector and insurance provider groups. Managed care programs became popular when private corporations and industry affiliations took an active part in maintaining control over soaring health care expenditures (Federation of American Health Systems Review, 1988).

Medical case management has become an effective way for private industry groups to maintain control over the use and costs of health care and to develop effective management and intervention methods (Dentzer, 1991; Califano, 1987; Katz, 1991). Case management identifies procedures that are used excessively and involve extended length of hospital stays and evaluates health care delivery systems that lack coordination and promote duplication and fragmentation of services. Medical case management controls both the demand for and the supply of health care by identifying potential high-cost cases (appropriate targeting); coordinating and channeling the delivery of care among providers, patients, insurers, and agencies that may be involved; and evaluating and managing the patient's existing benefits plan to cover needed services (Dentzer, 1991; Henderson, Bergman, Collard, et al, 1987; Henderson & Collard, 1988).

Until recently, the cost-effectiveness of the case management method has not been implicitly justified. Past research investigations were concerned with process and structured measures of efficiency. Such investigations evaluated whether or not the use of a physician as a case manager or an HMO as an insurer and provider of care actually resulted in reduced health care expenditures and increased quality assurance (Austin, 1983; Manning, Liebowitz, Goldberg, et al, 1984).

In 1986, a major study was undertaken by researchers at the Bigel Institute for Health Policy Studies at Brandeis University. This 2-year project was supported by funding from The Robert Wood Johnson Foundation to evaluate medical case management for catastrophic illnesses (Henderson, Bergman, Collard, et al, 1987; Henderson & Collard, 1988; Henderson & Wallack, 1987). The project involved the evaluation of a case management program offered by a predominantly private insurance group and was representative of other case management arrangements offered by other major insurers (Henderson, Bergman, Collard, et al, 1987).

Patient case load was identified by five diagnostic categories, which included the high risk infant, head trauma, spinal cord injury, cancer, and AIDS (Henderson, et al, 1987; Henderson & Wallack, 1987). Cost criteria were developed that incorporated the economic rationale of limiting inappropriate use of high-cost procedures and unnecessary ancillary resources. The factors responsible for managing the expenditures of high-cost patients included patient length of stay that exceeded predefined limits, evidence of complications indicated by the primary and secondary diagnosis, a repeat admission within a set time frame, and total patient charges exceeding a certain limit (Henderson & Wallack, 1987).

Cost-effectiveness was determined when the case management program initiated and implemented an alternative plan that decreased the patient's length of stay in the hospital, facilitated patient transfer to a less costly facility, and decreased expenditures associated with home care services (Henderson, et al, 1987).

Case management responsibilities in this study were assigned to registered nurses who were accountable for the assessment, care planning, monitoring, and evaluation activities. A case management plan was developed that incorporated the input of the physician provider and used appropriate resources to meet the individual needs of the patient and family (Henderson & Collard, 1988). Henderson and Collard (1988) found that the successful implementation of the case management plan rested with the cooperation of the attending physician. For the most part, case management was seen as a comprehensive plan for ensuring patients would receive health care services that would not ordinarily be reimbursable.

The Brandeis study found that use of the medical case management model resulted in significant cost savings. Several factors were identified as contributing to the effectiveness of this program. These factors include the following:

1. Early patient identification and intervention assures access to the most appropriate and least restrictive care.
2. Appropriate resource use helps maintain cost-effective care.
3. Alternative treatment programming and benefit management allows for flexibility in the payment structure.
4. Directing of the case management approach to specific patient groups helps achieve significant gains from services.
5. A cooperative and supportive relationship develops between the care provider and case recipients.
6. Interpretable, standardized reporting mechanisms help relate program objectives to patient care delivery.
7. Case management integrates the case planning process with resource allocation based on a patient classification system or DRG methodology.
8. A computerized information system allows for continuous data monitoring and analysis (Henderson, et al, 1987; Henderson & Collard, 1988; Weisman, 1987; White, 1986).

CASE MANAGEMENT AND CATASTROPHIC ILLNESS

Case management models differ depending on the patient populations they serve. Such variation makes it possible to match a particular patient's needs with the appropriate case management approach. For example, the primary care case management model, when used for treating chronically ill patients, may require the addition of medical or social case management services (Merrill, 1985).

Although no one model of case management is applicable in all circumstances, medical case management programs have recently been adapted for use in the management of care associated with catastrophic illness or injury (Brown, 1988;

Henderson & Wallack, 1987). Traditionally, care of those with catastrophic illnesses has been expensive because of a lack of coordination and fragmentation of services. Duplication of patient services and failure to work out alternative care arrangements have also added to the cost of treating catastrophic illness (Henderson & Collard, 1987). The medical case management model focuses cost containment efforts on a small percentage of the patient population that contains frequent users of hospital and medical technology services (Rosenbloom & Gertman, 1984; Zook & Moore, 1980). Zook and Moore (1980) identified two types of catastrophic cases that used a considerable amount of health care resources. The first group consisted of unanticipated illnesses such as spinal cord injury, head trauma, neonatal complications, cancer, cardiac disease, and stroke. The second type of catastrophic illness includes chronic medical or psychiatric conditions.

The rationale behind using the medical case management model with catastrophic illness is based on a study by the Health Data Institute of the medical care patterns of major businesses in the United States. This investigation showed that in more than 1 million episodes of hospital care occurring between 1980 and 1983, there were consistent patterns of high-cost illness. This study revealed that a large proportion of health care costs were attributable to only 5% to 10% of health-insured individuals (Rosenbloom & Gertman, 1984). Because catastrophic illness occurs less frequently than ordinary ailments, cost containment efforts should be directed to some of these high-cost illnesses. The Health Data Institute study indicates that medical, social, and financial consequences of catastrophic illness and injury can be controlled through a systematic effort characteristic of the case management approach.

REFERENCES

Aaron, H. (1991). Choosing from the health care reform menu. *The Journal of American Health Policy, 1*(3), 23-27.

Altman, S.H., & Rodmin, M.A. (1988). Halfway competitive markets and ineffective regulation: The American health care system. *Journal of Health Politics, Policy and Law, 13*(2), 323-339.

Austin, C.D. (1983). Case management in long-term care: Options and opportunities. *Health and Social Work, 8*(1), 16-30.

Bell, N. (1991). From the trenches: Strategies that work. *Business and Health, 9*(5), 19-25.

Brown, R. (1988). Principles for a national health program: A framework for analysis and development. *The Milbank Quarterly, 66*(4), 573-617.

Califano, J. (1987). Guiding the forces of the health care revolution. *Nursing and Health Care 8*(7), 400-404.

Christensen, L. (1991). The highs and lows of PPOs. *Business and Health, 9*(9), 72-77.

Dalton, J. (1987). Alternative delivery systems and employers. *Topics in Health Care Financing, 13*(3), 68-76.

Davis, R.G. (1985). Congress and the emergence of public health policy. *Health Care Management Review, 10*(1), 61-73.

Dentzer, S. (1991, September 23). Agenda for business: How to fight killer health costs. *U.S. News and World Report,* 50-58.

Dwyer, P., & Garland, S. (1991, November 25). A roar of discontent: Voters want health care reform now. *Business Week,* 28-30.

Eckholm, E. (1991, May 2). Rescuing health care. *The New York Times,* A 1, B 12.

Enthoven, A., & Kronick, R. (1989a). A consumer-choice health plan for the 1990s, part I. *New England Journal of Medicine, 320*(1), 29-37.

Enthoven, A., & Kronick, R. (1989b). A consumer-choice health plan for the 1990s, part II. *New England Journal of Medicine, 320*(2), 94-101.

Federation of American Health Systems Review (1988, July/August). Special report: The facts of life about managed care. Author, 20-49.

Frieden, J. (1991). Many roads lead to health system reform. *Business and Health, 9*(11), 38-66.

Garland, S. (1991, October 7). The health care crises: A prescription for reform. *Business Week,* 59-66.

Gilman, T., & Bucco, C. (1987). Alternate delivery systems: An overview. *Topics in Health Care Financing, 13*(3), 1-7.

Ginsburg, R.B., & Hackbarth, G.M. (1986). Alternative delivery systems and medicare. *Health Affairs, 5*(1), 6-22.

Henderson, M., Bergman, A., Collard, A., Souder, B., Wallack, S. (Draft, May 1, 1987). *Private sector medical case management for high cost illness.* Brandeis University Heller Graduate School Health Policy Center, Waltham, Massachusetts.

Henderson, M.G., & Wallack, S.S. (1987). Evaluating case management for catastrophic illness. *Business and Health, 4*(3), 7-11.

Henderson, M.G., & Collard, A. (1988). Measuring quality in medical case management programs. *Quality Review Bulletin, 14*(2), 33-39.

Herzlinger, R.E., & Schwartz, J. (1985). How companies tackle health care costs: Part I. *Harvard Business Review, 63*(4), 68-81.

Herzlinger, R.E. (1985). How companies tackle health care costs: Part II. *Harvard Business Review, 63*(5), 108-120.

Herzlinger, R.E., & Calkins, D. (1986). How companies tackle health care costs: Part III. *Harvard Business Review, 64*(1), 70-80.

Hewitt Associates. (1989). *Salaried employee benefits provided by major U.S. employers.* Lincolnshire, Ill.: Hewitt Associates.

Hicks, L., Stallmeyer, J., & Coleman, J. (1992). Nursing challenges in managed care. *Nursing Economics, 10*(4), 265-275.

Hospitals (1988, April 5). Managed care: Whoever has the data wins the game. *Hospitals,* 50-55.

Hospitals (1992, January 20). Health care reform a priority in the legislative years. *Hospitals,* 32-50.

Jones, K. (1989). Evolution of the prospective payment system: Implications for nursing. *Nursing Economics, 7*(6), 299-305.

Katz, F. (1991). Making a case for case management. *Business and Health, 9*(4), 75-77.

Kramon, G. (1989, January 8). Taking a scalpel to health costs. *The New York Times,* pp. 1, 9.

Luft, H.S. (1978). How do health maintenance organizations achieve their savings? Rhetoric and evidence. *New England Journal of Medicine, 298*(11), 1336-1343.

Luft, H.S. (1982). Health maintenance organizations and the rationing of medical care. *The Milbank Quarterly, 60*(2), 268-306.

Manning, W.G., Leibowitz, A., Goldberg, G., Rogers, W., & Newhouse, J. (1984). A controlled trial of the effect of a prepaid group practice on the use of services. *New England Journal of Medicine, 310*(23), 1505-1510.

Merrill, J.C. (1985). Defining case management. *Business and Health, 3*(5-9), 5-9.

Mullen, P. (1988, December 27). Big increase in health premiums. *Health Week, 2*(26), 1, 26.

National League for Nursing (1991). *Nursing's agenda for health care reform.* New York, N.Y.: NLN.

O'Connor, K. (1991). Risky business: HMOs and managed care. *Business and Health, 9*(6), 30-34.

Peres, A. (1992). Business must act now to shape reform. *Business and Health, 10*(1), 72.

Reinhardt, U.E. (1987a, January 11). Toward a fail-safe health-insurance system. *The Wall Street Journal.*

Reinhardt, U.E. (1987b). Health insurance for the nation's poor. *Health Affairs, 6*(1), 101-102.

Rosenberg, S., Perlis, H., Lynne, D., & Leto, L. (1991). A second look at second surgical opinions. *Business and Health, 9*(2), 14-28.

Rosenbloom, D., & Gertman, P. (1984). An intervention strategy for controlling costly care. *Business and Health, 1*(8), 17-21.

Sloan, F., Morrisey, M., & Valvona, J. (1988). Effects of the medicare prospective payment system on hospital cost containment: An early appraisal. *The Milbank Quarterly, 66*(2), 191-220.

Sloss, E.M., Keeler, E.B., Brook, R.H., Operskalski, B.H., Goldberg, G.A., & Newhouse, J.P. (1987). Effect of a health maintenance organization on physiologic health. *Annals of Internal Medicine, 106*(1), 130-138.

Swoap, D. (1984). Beyond DRGs: Shifting the risk to providers. *Health Affairs, 3*(4), 117-121.

Tallon, J.R. (1991). A report from the front line: Policy and politics in health reform. *The Journal of American Health Policy, 1*(1), 47-50.

Thorpe, K. (1991). The national health insurance conundrum: Shifting paradigms and potential solutions. *The Journal of American Health Policy, 1*(1), 17-22.

Traska, M.R. (1989). What 1989 holds for health benefits. *Business and Health, 1*(1), 22-30.

Waldo, D.R., Levit, J.R., & Lazenby, H. (1986). National health expenditures, 1985. *Health Care Financing Review, 8*(1), 1-21.

Weisman, E. (1987). Practical approaches for developing a case management program. *Quality Review Bulletin, 13*(11), 380-382.

Welling, K. (1990, June 11). The sickening spiral: Health-care costs continue to grow at an alarming rate. *Barron's,* 8.

White, M. (1986). Case management. In G.L. Maddox (Ed.), *The Encyclopedia of Aging* (pp. 92-96). New York: Springer Publishing.

Wilensky, G. (1991). Treat the causes, not the symptoms of the health care cost problem. *The Journal of American Health Policy, 1*(2), 15-17.

Zook, C.V., & Moore, F.D. (1980). High-cost users of medical care. *New England Journal of Medicine, 302*(18), 996-1002.

Patient Mix and Cost Related to Length of Hospital Stay

CHAPTER OVERVIEW

Prospective payment systems have influenced the development of innovative care delivery models by placing limits on the use of hospital resources. Because the length of time an individual spends in the hospital affects the appropriation of services and costs involved in that care, the number of hospitalized days becomes a very important variable in assessing and measuring the institution's financial outcome.

Numerous variables have been evaluated regarding their effects on the cost and length of stay of hospitalized patients. These variables include age, gender, diagnosis, comorbidity, discharge planning, patient care delivery models, and organizational factors.

The effects of care delivery models on health care services provided an important strategy for evaluating system effectiveness, efficiency, and quality. The coordination and integration required for case management are two reasons why such a health care delivery model maximizes the use and allocation of available resources and services.

Nursing case management methods provide indicators that help assess the effectiveness of patient care delivery. By focusing on the coordination and integration of inpatient services, nursing case management can reduce the patient length of stay while keeping it within medically appropriate boundaries.

With the implementation of DRG strategies, patient length of stay has become an overall indicator of a hospital's financial performance and cost-effectiveness. Numerous variables that have an effect on the cost and length of stay have been identified. This section will review and analyze studies related to patient length-of-stay variables.

The following section will be divided into three general categories. The first category will include patient demographics, for example, age and gender variables. The second category will include related variables, such as diagnosis and comorbidity, discharge planning, patient care delivery systems, and nursing intensity and workload. A critique of the nursing intensity and workload studies is provided. The third category will relate some of the nonclinical variables that affect patient length of stay. These variables include day-of-the-week admission (weekday versus weekend) and organizational factors.

PATIENT DEMOGRAPHICS

Certain patient characteristics, such as age, were reported to be important in judging the postoperative recovery time of patients undergoing surgical procedures, such as a hernia repair or a cholecystectomy (Kolouch, 1965). Although the reasons for a correlation between age and length of surgical convalescent time were not provided, the finding was anticipated because of the close association between age, chronicity, hospital-induced infections, age-related risk factors, patient dependency needs, and increased time required for postoperative healing.

In this study, however, age did not account for all of the variations in average length of stay reported by surgical case mix. Other variables existed that were not subject to control such as postoperative surgical complications, patient rehabilitation time, method of payment (i.e. third-party, Blue Cross, or charity), and type of hospital (i.e. teaching or nonteaching).

In another study by Marchette and Holloman (1986), age was the significant variable in prolonging the length of stay of cerebral vascular accident (CVA) patients. On average, the CVA patients were older and had the longest hospital stays. Again, as in the Kolouch (1965) study, age did not account for all of the diversity attributed to length of stay. Other intervening variables, such as severity of illness, discharge planning, and social consults, also affected the average length of stay of the hospitalized patients.

Posner and Lin (1975) studied the age variable in association with predicted length of stay for medical patients. In this study, age was evaluated in terms of its effects on comparable diagnoses. The study also evaluated the effect of various hospital settings (voluntary or municipal) on the length of patient stay. It was found that the hospital length of stay was not exclusively affected by the age of the patient. Wide variations were found in length of stay within age groups even when diagnostic categories and hospital variables were controlled.

The unreliability of age as a predictor of hospital length of stay was confirmed in another study by Lave and Leinhardt (1976). This study placed emphasis on case-mix factors and variables that related to the patient's medical condition and that contributed to changes in the patient's length of stay.

Both Lave and Leinhardt (1976) and Marchette and Holloman (1986) looked at the effect of gender on patient length of stay. Findings showed that male patients have shorter lengths of hospital stay than female patients and that single women have the longest stays. Several explanations of these findings were offered. First, because women live longer than men, women will experience more hospitalizations. Second, single women have longer stays because they have less availability of other adult family members to care for them. Although all of these findings are associated with longer than average hospital stays, the effect of patient gender could not be validated. Lave and Leinhardt (1976) advised that although patient demographic variables may be statistically significant in some situations, such variables may have a very minimal effect on the overall variability of the patient's length of stay.

CLINICALLY RELATED VARIABLES

The patient's primary diagnosis, number of surgical procedures, and the number of secondary diagnoses were factors that had a significant effect on patient length of stay (Lave & Leinhardt, 1976; Lew, 1966; McCorkle, 1970; Ro, 1969). These variables were found to account for 38% of the variation in length of stay, with primary diagnosis alone accounting for 27% of the variability in patient length of stay (Lave & Leinhardt, 1976). Patients diagnosed with acute myocardial infarction had the longest hospital stays, whereas patients with hyperplasia of the prostate had shorter lengths of stay. The findings indicate that patients with urgent or emergent status had longer hospital stays. In addition, the poor health condition of such patients on admission and the unscheduled nature of these admissions resulted in delays and inefficient mobilization of hospital services.

In two earlier studies, Riedel and Fitzpatrick (1964) and Mughrabi (1976) concluded that the primary diagnosis and the concomitant levels of severity are the most important factors contributing to the length of a patient's hospitalization. Additional studies indicated that comorbidity and/or related complications resulted in significantly longer lengths of stay (Berki, Ashcraft & Newbrander, 1984; Grau & Kovner, 1986).

In an investigation conducted by Marchette and Holloman (1986) both nurses' and social workers' discharge planning was found to affect patient length of stay. This study demonstrated a decrease of 0.8 days of hospitalization for those patients who received discharge planning early in their hospital stays. Conversely, the length of stay increased by 0.8 days for those patients who received discharge planning later in their hospitalization. In addition, a decrease of 2 days of hospitalization was shown because of nurses' discharge planning activities with patients diagnosed with CVA. This finding demonstrates that the effect of discharge planning is indicative of individual patient diagnoses (Cable & Mayers, 1983).

Timely social service planning and early referral programs were shown to shorten a patient's length of stay. Factors associated with changes in patients' Medicaid status, a lack of alternate care resources, noncompliance of medical staff to complete transfer and referral forms, and other confounding variables resulted in a delay of patient discharge.*

The nursing case management model for patient care delivery has been recognized for its significant effect on decreasing patient length of stay (Zander, 1988). Through the coordination and monitoring of resources needed for patient care, ischemic stroke patients' length of stay was reduced by 29%, and adult

---

*Altman, 1965; Zimmer, 1974; Schuman, Ostfeld & Willard, 1976; Schrager, Halman, Myers, Nichols & Rosenblum, 1978; Boone, Coulton & Keller, 1981; Farren, 1991.

leukemia patients' length of stay decreased from an average of 6 to 8 weeks to 32 days.

Rogers (1992) makes a distinction between the way that beyond-the-walls and within-the-walls models affect length of stay.

> Both models involve nurses in relatively autonomous positions that use a holistic nursing approach, "system savvy," collaboration to coordinate professional care team functions, and individualized care planning to achieve reductions in resource utilization while enhancing actual, as well as perceived, quality of care. The reduction in patient anxiety and increased patient compliance when they are more involved in the process and assured that someone they know is watching over things is attested to almost daily. These translate to reduced demands on nursing time during a given stay and in reductions in the actual length of stay.
>
> Beyond this, our experience has been that enhanced transit through the course of a stay and improved discharge planning, particularly with acute cases, takes days off of the end of the stay. This phenomena is a hallmark of the WTW model.
>
> On the other hand, the forte of the BTW models is care of the chronically ill. The impact of these models on LOS tends to be on the beginning of the stay. This occurs because the BTW nurse case managers know their patients' patterns and disease processes very well. They tend to get these patients into the hospital earlier in an exacerbation than they previously were. Being admitted "less sick" tends to keep these patients out of high-cost emergency and critical care departments and keep the overall LOS down. This phenomena was noted by Ethridge and Lamb (1989); and alluded to by Rogers, et al (1991). St. Joseph Medical Center in Wichita, in an unpublished internal management analyses, has since documented an overall reduction in the admission acuity for their BTW patients."

A major problem with studies relating to patient care delivery systems is the lack of uniformity and sophistication in defining costs. Variations exist as to what factors should be included in direct and indirect cost categories. Some studies included supplies and equipment, while other investigations allocated costs based on overhead expenses from ancillary and support services and general hospital operations. In some studies, nursing costs included the professional services of registered nurses. In other studies, nursing costs included all of the costs of providing nursing care to hospitalized patients (Edwardson & Giovannetti, 1987). Further research is needed to determine the applicability of cost accounting approaches to nursing models of care with the expected clinical and financial outcomes.

Nursing intensity, which is the amount of nursing care provided per patient day, along with various nursing interventions and staffing levels, was cited as reducing length of stay and costs associated with hospitalization. In an investigation done by Halloran (1983a, 1983b), nursing diagnoses were used to classify patients according to their nursing care requirements and to describe the time spent by professional nurses in caring for patients. Nursing diagnoses describe patient conditions and problems that require nursing intervention. It was found that a predominantly registered nurse staff versus a staffing mix of registered nurses, licensed practical nurses, and nursing attendants, resulted in decreased costs associated with patient care. The investigation showed that an all-registered-nurse staff would be more likely to deal with total patient needs than a staff composed of various skill mixes. Halloran also proposed that nursing care costs should be identified and defined according to nursing diagnoses (unit of service) instead of the medical DRG currently in use.

In another study, Halloran and Kiley (1984) proposed a nursing information system model that allocated staffing and resources using nursing diagnoses. This process was based on a nursing workload unit of analysis that calculated costs using a patient classification system for staffing. The reason for using a patient classification system was that such a system made it possible to measure the nursing workload and allocate costs in order to distinguish the costs of nursing care services from the cost of the hospital's room and board rate.

As outlined by Edwardson and Giovannetti (1987), the patient classification system makes it possible to calculate the hours of care used during a patient's hospitalization. Once the number of patient care hours is identified, this number is translated into a dollar amount. Patients are then classified into DRG categories, and nursing care costs for patients are aggregated and analyzed.

Although patient classification systems offer a more reliable representation than traditional methods of identifying the nursing care needs of patients (i.e., global averages, such as the average amount of care required per day by the typical patient), there are still some inherent problems. As identified by Giovannetti (1972) and Edwardson and Giovannetti (1987) the problems associated with this system include the inadvisability of comparing a patient classification system developed in one hospital with that in another because of the differences in treatment modalities, architectural structure and design of the inpatient units, and standards and policies of the institution. Some of the factors used to weigh the categories are subjective, which results in problems of reliability. Furthermore, methods of validating the system and workload indexes are not transferable. In spite of these difficulties, the method of staffing by workload index has been a generally accepted mode by health care institutions across the country.

An investigation done by Halloran and Halloran (1985) found that nursing diagnoses were accurate for predicting nursing workload and quantity of nursing care. In addition, nursing diagnoses contributed to some of the variation in patient length of stay. It was suggested that nursing instead of medical needs kept patients in the hospital. Nursing diagnoses that dealt with the patient's psychosocial needs and self-care requirements were found to be significant in increasing nursing workload. In another study, nursing workload activities correlated with 77% of the patient's length of hospitalization. These findings imply that variations in length of stay within specific DRG categories can be explained by the clinical management of patient care by nurses (Halloran & Kiley, 1986).

Ventura, Young, Feldman, Pastore, Pikula, and Yates (1985) found that nursing interventions associated with health protection activities for patients with peripheral vascular disease significantly decreased the patient's length of stay and lowered hospitalization costs, which were based on a fixed per diem rate. Mumford, Schlesinger and Glass (1982) and Devine and Cook (1983) demonstrated that psychologic and educational interventions (i.e. patient teaching related to pain prevention and complications) with postsurgical patients reduced the length of stay and improved patient recovery time.

Flood and Diers (1988) identified the effect of professional nurse staffing levels on length of stay. According to the study, decreased nurse staffing levels could lead to a reduction in productivity and inadequate patient care resulting in longer hospitalization. Patients whose case mixes included gastrointestinal hemorrhages and CVAs and who had been located on a unit with significant staffing shortages were found to have longer lengths of stay, 3.80 and 4.14 days respectively, when compared with patients on a unit that had adequate staffing levels. The increase in length of stay was attributed to patient-related complications and nosocomial infections and resulted in the use of high levels of nursing care resources.

However, the findings of the Flood and Diers study are speculative, because many of the variables associated with patient length of stay, for example, primary diagnosis, comorbidity, medical complications, and discharge planning factors, had not been controlled. Because these variables were not controlled, the study is not adequate for showing a significant correlation between nurse staffing levels and length of stay.

The results of the nursing intensity and workload investigations support the premise that patient care requirements, nursing interventions, and level of staff affect the delivery of care. However, other variables, that have a profound effect on the delivery of nursing care services were not accounted for. Some of these variables were identified by Edwardson and Giovannetti (1987) and include service standards of the institution, physician practice patterns, nature and extent of support services, adequacy of the physical plant, and quality-of-care indexes. The last variable would have to be studied with various mixes of staffing personnel to determine the efficacy of patient care delivery.

The general findings of the nursing intensity and workload studies take on a different perspective when viewed in light of the investigations done by the Prospective Payment Assessment Commission (ProPAC). ProPAC was established as an independent advisory board to the Department of Health and Human Services (HHS) and Congress to report on issues surrounding the impact of the prospective payment system on health care delivery and finance. ProPAC's responsibilities include annual recommendations to HHS regarding appropriate changes in Medicare payments for inpatient hospital care and changes in the relative weights of DRGs. ProPAC is also required to report to Congress its evaluation of any adjustments made to DRG classifications and weights (Price & Lake, 1988).

ProPAC focused its research efforts on the DRG allocation method as it related to the intensity of nursing care. The nursing intensity and workload studies done over the last few years established that inaccuracies existed in the allocation of DRG weights to nursing costs. In the past, nursing service in health care institutions was calculated as part of the room and board rate and did not directly affect patient charges. Variations in the patient's nursing care and attributable costs were strictly related to the patient's length of stay and routine and intensive care levels (Cromwell & Price, 1988; Young, 1986).

Accounting for the amount of time spent and for the type of care delivered by nursing is one problem generated by the nature of the services offered. Defining nursing care through a patient classification system became one way of alleviating this difficulty. Matching the type of care a patient will need with a specific category on the patient classification instrument and then determining the amount of nursing resources needed for that patient category provided the foundation for establishing the costs of nursing services and developing a basis for charges to patients. The patient classification system was used as an instrument to measure the severity level of patients (in terms of nursing workload) as well as variations in nursing care. However, studies have shown that because of systematic errors (i.e., quantity of care and level of care are both objective and subjective estimates), a lack of cross-institutional comparability and generalizability, and lack of on-going validity and reliability, patient classification systems were not accurate resources for determining the cost of nursing services (Dijkers & Paradise, 1986). In addition, the wide variations in the methodologies used in the numerous nursing intensity studies question the appropriateness and applicability of using nursing patient classification systems to account for DRG-specific nursing intensity values (Price & Lake, 1988).

In view of these limitations, a major research effort directed by ProPAC to provide national adjustments of DRG weights based on nursing intensity variations was abandoned (Cromwell & Price, 1988; Price & Lake, 1988). Recommendations from ProPAC for further research included:

- Developing nursing intensity adjustments for selected DRGs on a case-by-case basis
- Documenting nursing intensity variation with DRGs over a patient's length of stay by identifying factors related to patient complexity, changes in staff volume, and skill mix
- Establishing uniformity among patient classification systems
- Establishing the cost base used to allocate DRG weights

ProPAC also said that the effects of nursing intensity on DRG weights would be greater if applied to all routine and department costs rather than just direct nursing care (Cromwell & Price, 1988; Price & Lake, 1988).

NONCLINICAL VARIABLES

Lew (1966) studied how the day of the week that a patient was admitted affected the average length of stay. Patients who came in for medical admissions on Sunday had the lowest average length of stay, 10.83 days, and those admitted on Friday had the highest average length of stay, 13.81 days. For surgical patients, those admitted on Wednesday had the lowest average length of stay, 9.88 days while those admitted on Friday had the highest average length of stay, 11.85 days. When medical and surgical admissions were combined, those patients admitted on Friday had the highest average length of stay while those admitted on Sunday had the lowest average length of stay. Reasons for the variations in the lengths of weekday stay were attributed to the availability of resources—such as personnel, operating rooms, equipment, and procedures—and services needed for the care of the patient.

Day-of-the-week variables were found significant in studies conducted by Lave and Leinhardt (1976) and Mughrabi (1976). However, these variables did not account for a large portion of the variation in average length of stay.

Institutional practices related to management, patient care delivery, and use of facility resources (e.g. laboratory, radiology) were among the many variables that affected length of stay. Becker, Shortell and Neuhouser (1980) identified managerial and organizational factors that had significant effects on overall patient length of stay. In this study, reductions in patient length of stay and increases in the quality and efficiency of hospital services were attributable to the following variables:

- Awareness of the administrative and clinical managers of traditional outcome measurements of patient care (i.e., length of stay, infection and mortality indexes, and preventable complications) compared with other hospitals
- The degree of professional autonomy related to hospital operations and clinical decision-making
- Interdisciplinary as well as interdepartmental collaboration and accountability for the efficient use, coordination, and monitoring of hospital resources including nursing services, radiology, and laboratory

Decreased length of hospital stay facilitated by interdepartmental coordination and integration of patient services was achieved by the using regularly scheduled meetings among radiology, nursing service, and laboratory personnel.

Another study, conducted by Berki, Ashcraft, and Newbrander (1984), showed that with certain DRG classifications, patient length-of-stay variations were related to use and consumption of hospital services. Increases in laboratory and radiology services were found to be associated with longer lengths of stay in those DRG categories, such as diabetes and arthritis, that required intensive use of ancillary services. Other DRG categories—for example, eye disease, which requires reattachment of the retina and repair of the cornea,—increased nursing service intensity and resulted in decreased patient length of stay.

REFERENCES

Altman, I. (1965). Some factors affecting hospital length of stay. *Hospitals, 39*(7), 68-176.

Becker, S., Shortell, S., & Neuhouser, D. (1980). Management practices and hospital length of stay. *Inquiry, 17*, 318-330.

Berki, S., Ashcraft, M., & Newbrander, W. (1984). Length of stay variations within ICDA-8 diagnosis related groups. *Medical Care, 22*(2), 126-142.

Boone, C., Coulton, C., & Keller, S. (1981). The impact of early and comprehensive social work services on length of stay. *Social Work in Health Care, 7*(1), 1-9.

Cable, E., & Mayers, S. (1983). Discharge planning effect on length of hospital stay. *Archives of Physical Medicine and Rehabilitation, 64*(2), 57-60.

Cromwell, J., & Price, K. (1988). The sensitivity of DRG weights to variation in nursing intensity. *Nursing Economics, 6*(1), 18-26.

Devine, E., & Cook, T. (1983). A meta-analytic analysis of effects of psychoeducational interventions on length of postsurgical hospital stay. *Nursing Research, 32*(5), 267-274.

Dijkers, M., & Paradise, T. (1986). PCS: One system for both staffing and costing. Do services rendered match need estimates? *Nursing Management, 17*(1), 25-34.

Edwardson, S., & Giovannetti, P. (1987). A review of cost accounting methods for nursing services. *Nursing Economics, 5*(3), 107-117.

Ethridge, P., & Lamb, G. (1989). Professional nursing case management improves quality, access and costs. *Nursing Management, 20*(3), 30-35.

Farren, E., (1991). Effects of early discharge planning on length of hospital stay. *Nursing Economics, 9*(1), 25-30.

Flood, S., & Diers, D. (1988). Nurse staffing, patient outcome and cost. *Nursing Management, 19* (5), 34-43.

Giovannetti, P. (May 1972). *Measurement of patient's requirements for nursing services.* Paper presented to the National Institute of Health Conference, Virginia.

Grau, L., & Kovnor, C. (1986). Comorbidity one length of stay: A case study. In F.A. Shaffer (Ed.), *Patients and purse strings: Patient classification and case management* (pp. 233-242). New York: National League for Nursing.

Halloran, E. (1983a). Staffing assignment: By task or by patient. *Nursing Management, 14*(8), 16-18.

Halloran, E. (1983b). RN staffing: More care less cost. *Nursing Management, 14*(9), 18-22.

Halloran, E. & Halloran, D. (1985). Exploring the DRG/nursing equation. *American Journal of Nursing, 85*(10), 1093-1095.

Halloran, E., & Kiley, M. (1984). Case mix management. *Nursing Management, 15*(2), 39-45.

Halloran, E., & Kiley, M.L. (1986). The nurse's role and length of stay. *Medical Care, 23*(9), 1122-1124.

Kolouch, F. (1965). Computer shows how patient stays vary. *The Modern Hospital, 105*(5), 130-134.

Lave, J., & Leinhardt, S. (1976). The cost and length of a hospital stay. *Inquiry, 13,* 327-343.

Lew, I. (1966). Day of the week and other variables affecting hospital admissions, discharges and length of stay for patients in the Pittsburgh area. *Inquiry, 3,* 3-39.

Marchette, L., & Holloman, F. (1986). Length of stay variables. *Journal of Nursing Administration, 165*(3), 12-19.

McCorkle, L. (1970). Duration of hospitalization prior to surgery. *Health Services Research, 5,* 114-131.

Mughrabi, M.A. (1976). The effects of selected demographic and clinical variables on the length of hospital stay. *Hospital Administration in Canada, 18,* 82-88.

Mumford, E., Schlesinger, H. & Glass, G. (1982). The effects of psychological intervention on recovery from surgery and heart attacks: An analysis of the literature. *American Journal of Public Health, 72*(2), 141-151.

Posner, J., & Lin, H. (1975). Effects of age on length of hospital stay in a low income population. *Medical Care, 13*(10), 855-875.

Price, K., & Lake, E. (1988). ProPAC's assessment of DRGs and nursing intensity. *Nursing Economics, 6*(1), 10-16.

Riedel, D., & Fitzpatrick, T. (1964). *Patterns of patient care: A study of hospital use in six diagnosis.* Ann Arbor: The University of Michigan Graduate School of Business Administration.

Ro, K.K. (1969). Patient characteristics, hospital characteristics and hospital use. *Medical Care, 7*(4), 295-312.

Rogers, M., Personal communication. (August 1992).

Rogers, M., Riordan, J., & Swindle, D. (1991). Community-based nursing case management pays off. *Nursing Management, 22*(3), 30-34.

Schrager, J., Halman, M., Myers, D., Nichols, R., & Rosenblum, L. (1978). Impediments to the course and effectiveness of discharge planning. *Social Work in Health Care, 4*(1), 65-79.

Schuman, J., Ostfeld, A., & Willard, H. (1976). Discharge planning in an acute hospital. *Archives of Physical Medicine and Rehabilitation, 57*(7), 343-347.

Ventura, M., Young, D., Feldman, M.J., Pastore, P., Pikula, S., & Yates, M.A. (1985). Cost savings as an indicator of successful nursing intervention. *Nursing Research, 34*(1), 50-53.

Young, D. (1986). ProPAC: Future Directions. *Nursing Economics, 4*(1), 12-15.

Zander, K. (1988). Nursing care management: Strategic management of cost and quality outcomes. *Journal of Nursing Administration, 18*(5), 23-30.

Zimmer, J. (1974). Length of stay and hospital bed misutilization. *Medical Care, 12*(5), 453-462.

10

Policy and Legislation

CHAPTER OVERVIEW

Because the prospective payment system gave hospitals the incentive to shorten length of stay, strategies using case management are being developed to focus on postdischarge planning and community-based long-term care. Case management has also demonstrated its applicability as a resource in the development of health legislation and policy in regard to the delivery of patient care. The usefulness of case management is an integral part of the administration and management of health care and is also a vital cost containment measure.

HISTORICAL LEGISLATION

At present 37 states have Medicaid provisions for case management. Legislation for governing the practices of case managers and for developing national certification and specific state requirements is also pending. (National Case Management Task Force Steering Committee, 1992; Sager, 1992).

Case management has been integrated into many of the federal and state policies associated with the delivery of health care and social support services. The overall goal is to reduce the use and costs of expensive treatments. Case management is used in these situations to reduce institutionalization, increase and monitor access of needed services, and expand alternative community resources such as home and long-term care (Boling, 1992; Capitman, 1986; Kane, 1985; Strickland, 1992).

Case management has also been a major component in several federally funded demonstration projects.

The Triage demonstration project provided case management and health care services outside the traditional Medicare benefits. These services include adult day-care, companion homemaking services, counseling, transportation, pharmaceuticals, and access to residential care. Eligibility requirements included those individuals who were more than 65 years old and had medical, social, and financial problems; an increased likelihood for institutionalization; and a failing support system. Case management services were provided by a professional team consisting of registered nurses, physicians, and social workers (O'Rourke, Raisz & Segal, 1982).

People eligible for the Wisconsin Community Care Organization included those individuals who were at risk for institutionalization as determined by the Geriatric Functional Rating Scale. This scale rated individuals' ability to perform functional and cognitive activities.

Services included companion and home-health-aide services, medical supplies and equipment, transportation, respite care, and skilled nursing care (Applebaum, Seidl & Austin, 1980; Seidl, Applebaum, Austin & Mahoney, 1983).

The On Lok demonstration project provided case management to dependent and elderly individuals eligible for skilled nursing or intermediate nursing home care. Acute care services, including hospitalization, were also provided in addition to other services. These other services included adult and social day-care, dental care, home health care, optometry, and occupational and pharmaceutical services. Case management is provided by registered nurses, physicians, social workers, physical and occupational therapists, and dietitians (Zawadski, Shen, Yordi & Hansen, 1984).

The New York City Home Care program offered services to chronically ill and elderly individuals residing in the New York City area. The program provided homemaker and personal care, transportation assistance, and various medical therapies (Sainer, Brill, Horowitz, et al, 1984).

The Long-Term Care Channeling Demonstration Project provided case management services to dependent and chronically ill individuals. Services included mental health counseling, homemaking, personal care, supportive services, such as adult foster care and day-care, skilled nursing, transportation, medical therapies, and equipment (Applebaum, Harrigan & Kemper, 1986; Kemper et al, 1986; Wooldridge & Schore, 1986).

Those who were eligible for Access, Medicare's long-term care demonstration project, included all individuals 18 or older and Medicare beneficiaries older than 65 who needed long-term, skilled nursing care. Services ranged from case management, skilled nursing and home care, and Medicaid-waived services. Waived services included community health nursing, home health aide, medical and nursing consultations and therapies, personal care, equipment and supplies, respite care, and transportation (Berkeley Planning Associates, 1987; Eggert, Bowlyow & Nichols, 1980).

CURRENT LEGISLATION AFFECTING HEALTH CARE

Recent legislation and health care reform proposals point to principles of managed or coordinated care for providing a framework for cost-effective health care delivery. By focusing on case management and long-term care, an alternative to costly hospital and institutional care can be found. These legislative proposals seek to reduce unneeded care and the use of expensive inpatient services through preventive and primary care interventions. They also support comprehensive community-based services and initiatives to improve overall health status and prevent inappropriate hospitalizations (Blankenau, 1992; Pollack, 1992; Strickland, 1992; Wagner, 1991).

Targeted populations include, among others, the chronically ill elderly, young and middle-age individuals with chronic illness and disabilities, the uninsured, and the impoverished. Resources also will be directed to reducing infant mortality and improving maternal health status (Darman, 1991; Hospitals, 1992a; Wagner, 1991).

Managed care is playing a major role in proposals to expand Medicaid. *Managed Medicaid* legislation, passed in 1987, makes recommendations for a flat payment for Medicaid beneficiaries in need of medical and long-term care. This plan reduces hospital stays and excessive use of services, increases affordable access, and strengthens community-based services and resources (Hospitals, 1992b; McNeil, 1991; "Medicaid-Mandated Managed Care," 1992).

Another example of how the concept of case managed care is used is with the recent legislation of the CHAMPUS (Civilian Health and Medical Program of the Uniformed Services) Reform Initiative (CRI). This plan extends coverage under a case managed structure for military dependents and retirees younger than 65 (Burke, 1992). It also helps reduce health care expenditures and increase access by encouraging the use of military medical services and facilities (Burke, 1992).

Of the major reform plans being introduced, six address long-term care policies and legislation. It is important to note that these health reform proposals represent the harbinger of legislation for case management. The proposals are currently being debated and are pending legislation by Congress within the year.

The Pepper Commission Proposal, developed by the Bipartisan Commission on Health Care, extends Medicare's long-term care initiatives to all disabled individuals. Under the proposal, which was introduced in the Senate by Senator Jay Rockefeller (D-W.Va.), eligibility will be determined by state, local, or federally funded agencies and will be based on standardized assessments of the beneficiary's resources and support systems.

Case managers will be used to evaluate and monitor the services provided. Benefits include comprehensive home- and community-based services that involve skilled nursing; physical, occupational, and speech therapies; personal care; homemaker services; adult and social day care; respite care for caregivers; hospital care; primary and preventive care; and support counseling (Darman, 1991; Harrington, 1990; Pepper Commission, 1990).

Coverage structure incorporates a play or pay plan that requires employers to provide health insurance to employees and their dependents or pay into a public tax plan. A provision is made in this plan for the phasing in of small businesses. Federal and state financing will be available to cover home- and community-based care programs and nursing-home care.

Quality-of-care issues are addressed through standardized practice guidelines, outcome research, and peer review. Overall costs for this proposal include $24 billion for home care and $18.8 billion for nursing home care (Darman, 1991; Frieden, 1991).

The Long-Term Home Care Act (HR 2263), introduced by Senator Claude Pepper (D-Fla.), provides coverage for the chronically ill or disabled elderly and children younger than 19 who have cognitive and functional impairments. It also includes individuals with severe functional disabilities.

Benefits include skilled nursing care, homemaker and personal care services, physical, occupational, speech, and respiratory therapies, medical supplies and equipment, caregiver education, support and counseling, and adult day-care. Eligibility determination is made by a long-term care management agency or private nonprofit agency along with the individual's physician.

Patient care management is provided through case management agencies that do not have affiliations or control interest in the referral facilities. Estimated costs for this plan are at $8.9 billion for 1993 (Darman, 1991).

The Elder Care Program (HR 3140), proposed by Representative Harry Waxman (D-CA), provides for Medicare beneficiaries and disabled individuals. Eligibility determination is made by community assessment and review agencies that are restricted in affiliation and ownership to community or nursing care facilities.

Home and community-based services include adult day-care, skilled nursing, homemaker and personal-care services, medical and social services, diagnostic tests, medical supplies and equipment, caregiver education and training, and physical and occupational therapies. Estimated costs range from $50 billion to $60 billion in 1992 (Darman, 1991; Hospitals, 1992a).

Life Care (S2163/HR4093), sponsored by Senator Edward Kennedy (D-Mass.) and Representative Edward Roybal (D-Calif.), extends eligibility to the chronically ill who are older than 65 or younger than 19, all disabled and dependent individuals, and people with a life expectancy of one year or less.

Eligibility determination and patient management is made by federally funded case management agencies. Benefit coverage includes up to the first 6 months of nursing home care with extended nursing home coverage provided through a federal long-term care insurance program.

Financial structure includes Medicaid and income-related subsidies. Services provided include skilled nursing, adult day-care, primary and preventive care, transportation to health and social care facilities, respite care, institutional or noninstitutional care, nutrition and dietary counseling, and physical, occupational, and speech therapies. The estimated cost of such a program is expected to be $20 billion (Darman, 1991; Harrington, 1990; Hospitals, 1992a).

Similar to Life Care, the Comprehensive Health Care Plan (HR 4253) provides for the chronically ill who are older than 65 or younger than 19. The plan also provides for Medicare-eligible disabled individuals of all ages and insures those with a life expectancy of 1 year or less.

Eligibility and patient care is determined by federally funded case management agencies. Benefits include nursing home coverage and income assistance programs.

Home and community-based services include skilled nursing; physical, occupational, and speech therapies; homemaker services; medical and social work care; transportation; adult day-care and respite care; and counseling services. The estimated cost of this plan is $258 billion, which includes universal health care and preventive and long-term care provisions (Darman, 1991).

MediPlan (HR 5300), sponsored by representative Pete Stark (D-Calif.), will extend Medicare benefits to chronically ill and disabled individuals of all ages. This plan will also include primary and preventive care to children in addition to well-baby care.

Eligibility determination and patient management are conducted by case management agencies, which have provider and ownership restrictions. A full range of home- and community-based services are provided. These services include skilled nursing; counseling services; medical supplies; adult day-care; physical, occupational, and respiratory therapies; medical and social services; caregiver education and training; homemaker and personal care services; and prescription-drug coverage.

The plan's financing structure incorporates payroll tax increases and state contributions. The estimated cost of such a program is $120 billion, which includes universal health care provisions and long-term care arrangements (Darman, 1991; Frieden, 1991; Hospitals, 1992a).

Additional legislative initiatives indicate case management as an integral component of health care delivery and policy formation. This plan is one of several state assembly and senate bills that have been developed in California and affect case management (Kowlsen, 1991). An overview of three such bills follows.

California Assembly Bill 1341 provides for a 3-year demonstration project to provide case management to children at risk for abuse and neglect. Case management services would be provided by public health nurses. The goal of this project is to reduce shelter or foster care placement and decrease emergency room visits and hospitalizations among children.

California Senate Bill 1108 establishes the Primary Care Case Management Advisory Board as part of the California Department of Health Services. It also provides for the delivery of case management services for Medicaid-eligible individuals to promote and increase accessibility to affordable health care resources.

California Assembly Bill 14 would ratify primary health care coverage to all individuals. Cost containment strategies would include managed care principles such as case management.

REFERENCES

Applebaum, R., Seidl, F.W., & Austin, C.D. (1980). The Wisconsin community care organization: Preliminary findings from the Milwaukee experiment. *Gerontologist, 20*, 350-355.

Applebaum, R.A., Harrigan, M.N. & Kemper, P. (1986). *The evaluation of the national long-term care demonstration: Tables comparing channeling to other community care demonstrations.* Princeton, New Jersey: Mathematica Policy Research, Inc.

Berkeley Planning Associates (1987). *Evaluation of the Access: Medicare long-term care demonstration project. Final Report.* Berkeley, California.

Blankenau, R. (1992, January 6). Health-reform bills top 1992 agendas of Hill health leaders. *AHA News.*

Boling, J. (1992). An American integrated health care system? Where are we now? *The case manager, 3*(3), 53-59.

Burke, M. (1992, January 20). Armed services are marching toward managed care alternatives. *AHA News, 28*(3), pg. 6.

Capitman, J.A. (1986). Community-based long-term care models, target groups, and impacts on service use. *Gerontologist, 26*(4), 389-397.

Darman, R. (1991, October 10). *Comprehensive health reform: Observations about the problem and alternative approaches to solution. Presented to the House Committee on Ways and Means.* Washington, D.C.: Executive Office of the President, Office of Management and Budget.

Eggert, G., Bowlyow, J., & Nichols, C. (1980). Gaining control of the long-term care systems: First returns from the access experiment. *Gerontologist, 20,* 356-363.

Frieden, J. (1991). Many roads lead to health system reform. *Business and Health, 9*(11), 38-66.

Harrington, C. (1990). Policy options for a national health care plan. *Nursing Outlook, 38*(5), 223-228.

Hospitals (1992a, January 20). Health care reform a priority in the new legislative year. 32-50.

Hospitals (1992b, March 20). Managed care in the 1990s: Providers' new role for innovative health delivery. 26-34.

Kane, R. (1985). Case management in health care settings. In M. Weil & J. Karls (Eds.), *Case management in human service practice* (pp. 170-203). San Francisco: Josey Bass Pub.

Kemper, P., Brown, R., Carcagno, G., Applebaum, R., Christianson, J., Carson, W., Dunstan, S., Grannemann, T., Harrigan, M., Holden, N., Phillips, B., Schore, J., Thornton, C., Wooldridge, J., & Skidmore, F. (1986). *The evolution of the national long-term care demonstration: Final report.* Princeton, N.J.: Mathematica Policy Research, Inc.

Kowlsen, T. (1991, October). California dreaming. *Washington Health Beat,* 28-29.

McNeil, D. (1991, November 17). Washington tries to sort out health insurance proposals. *New York Times,* 2.

Medicaid-Mandated managed care. (1992, June). *Nursing & Health Care, 13*(6), p. 288.

National Case Management Task Force Steering Committee (1991-1992, February 9). *Work summary and survey of case management toward medical case manager certification.* Little Rock, Ark.: Systemedic Corporation.

O'Rourke, B., Raisz, H., & Segal, J. (1982). *Triage II: Coordinated delivery of services to the elderly: Final report.* Volume 1-2. Plainville, Conn.: Triage, Inc.

Pepper Commission (1990, March 2). Access to healthcare and long-term care for all Americans. Washington, D.C.: U.S. Bipartisan Commission on Comprehensive Health.

Pollack, R. (1992, January 13). Hospitals ready for reform of national health care system. *AHA News.*

Sager, O. (1992). Certification: From need to reality. *The Case Manager, 3*(3), 81-84.

Sainer, J.S., Brill, R.S., Horowitz, A., Weinstein, M., Dono, J.E., & Korniloff, N. (1984). *Delivery of medical and social services to the homebound elderly: A demonstration of intersystem coordination: Final report.* New York: New York City Department for the Aging.

Seidl, F.W., Applebaum, R., Austin, C., & Mahoney, K. (1983). *Delivering in-home services to the aged and disabled: The Wisconsin experiment.* Lexington, Mass.: Lexington Books.

Strickland, T. (1992, April, May, June). Profile [Interview with Gail R. Wilensky, Deputy Assistant to the President for Policy Development]. *The Case Manager, 3*(2), 72-81.

Wagner, L. (1991, December 9). Cost containment: Carrot or the stick? *Modern Healthcare,* 36-40.

Wooldridge, J., & Schore, J. (1986). *Evaluation of the national long-term care demonstration: Channeling effects on hospital, nursing home, and other medical services.* Princeton, N.J.: Mathematica Policy Research, Inc.

Zawadski, R.T., Shen, J., Yordi, C., & Hansen, J.C. (1984). *On Lok's community care organization for dependent adults: A research and development project (1978-1983): Final report.* San Francisco: On Lok Senior Health Services.

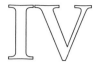

THE PLANNING PROCESS

11

Assessing the System and Creating an Environment for Change

CHAPTER OVERVIEW

Successful implementation of a case management system begins with a solid, well-conceived plan. The first step in creating the plan is to assess the system in which the case management model will be implemented. Human and financial resources should be reviewed. This information helps determine the degree of change that the organization can tolerate and the chances for a successful conversion.

Implementation involves a nine-step process. Target patient populations are identified and matched to nursing units and the design structure for the units is decided. This new structure involves a change in the staff mix. The next step is formation of interdisciplinary groups. These groups consist of the case manager, physician(s), social worker, and any other pertinent health care professionals. Benchmarks, which determine how the change will be monitored and evaluated over time, must be selected. Before implementation takes place, pre-implementation data must be collected. The next step involves educating staff, physicians and other professionals who will be affected by conversion to the case management model. At this stage training is provided for the case managers who will be required to function in their new roles. After managers are educated on how the model works it can be implemented. Finally, evaluation should take place at predetermined intervals. Necessary changes should be made as quickly as possible.

FEASIBILITY OF THE MODEL

Converting to a case management model requires systematic planning. A solid plan that has been well thought out guarantees a higher rate of successful conversion. Without a plan, it is likely that the expected outcome of the model will be lost or that some important elements will be left out.

Administrators have always known that a plan is essential for change in any organization. This philosophy is no less true for nurses attempting to create a major change such as a conversion to a case management model. The first step in any planning process is to determine if the change is not only feasible but also worthwhile. The potential for success and the effect such a change will have on the organization must be evaluated from both a positive and negative perspective. Overall the change should lead the organization in a positive direction.

ASSESSMENT OF RESOURCES

Assessing resources requires some homework. A thorough analysis of the organization, including its structure and financial status, needs to be done. Those implementing the change need to determine if the organization is strong enough to withstand the temporary instability that will accompany the change. As with any major change, errors will be made along the way. The complete support of all top administrators and a commitment to the long haul is absolutely necessary. In the beginning, the road will be a bumpy one, and everyone concerned should be aware of this and ready to be supportive every step of the way.

THE COST OF IMPLEMENTATION

A case management system can be implemented with few additional costs for the organization if the change is implemented carefully. For instance, when selecting units for the pilot program, choose units that have current openings or units that budgeted for an additional person. Such an opening can then be filled by someone qualified to be a case manager. In this way, the new position will not incur any costs outside of what was already budgeted. This is essential for a plan that must show success before it receives an allotment in the budget. Internal and preexisting resources can then be used for implementation.

If possible, the organization's budget should allow for certain expenditures needed for implementation. These expenditures will probably not be related to personnel costs unless the organization decides to hire a project manager. Costs may be incurred for documentation system changes or for data collection and/or statistical analysis necessary for measuring success.

Both administrative and financial support must be obtained before switching over to a case management system.

INTERNAL MARKETING

Obtaining the support of those in senior management is relatively easy if the administrators already have some familiarity with the model. Senior management may have heard or read about the model and already realized the need for such a change. Conversely, they may have misconceptions or may be misinformed about the model. Senior management might also object to the change solely because it comes at an inopportune time.

Senior management support is a prerequisite for beginning the change process. The ways in which the change may be attained will be as diverse as the management styles of the individuals involved. Making sure that administrators are familiar with those initiating the change and have positive working relationships with them will be essential for success.

Furthermore, the concept of the case management system should be introduced by someone who is familiar with the administrator, the president, the executive vice president of operations, the chief financial officer, or some other executive of the organization. Use of an outside consultant to introduce the concept is not advisable at this point. The individual who introduces the concept to the administrator must have the facts of implementation readily available. Estimated cost, staffing needs, and time-frames must be prepared for the first meeting. Expected outcomes, goals, and long-range plans should also be presented. A review of other organizations that have implemented the concept and have had positive results will lend credibility to the proposed plan.

It may be necessary to explain the definition of case management from a nursing perspective if the administrator has no previous knowledge of the model. Emphasis should be placed on how the model will benefit all disciplines. Finally, but possibly most important, is the need to review the financial implications of such a conversion. An initiative whose goal is to reduce patient length of stay may be the best-selling feature in today's financial climate. An explanation as to why a nurse may be best suited to monitor this process may take some extra effort. Many people believe that social work, utilization review, or the physicians themselves should be the facilitators and coordinators of the care plan. Other initiatives aimed at reducing length of stay may have already been attempted. The failure of these initiatives may help convince administrators to try a new approach. Do not fail to emphasize that, although nursing drives the process, all disciplines must take part in achieving success. The input and participation of all health care providers is an essential component, too. The keys to case management's success are both its nursing and interdisciplinary approach.

Within the prospective payment system, length of stay can determine financial success or failure. However, when discussing how case management affects a reduction in length of stay, the ways in which length of stay affects quality should also be emphasized. The cost/quality ratio as it relates to case management needs to be reviewed. Any initiative that reduces length of stay without looking at quality and resources, is doomed to fail the organization and the patients.

The support of nursing administration is another vital component. Nurse managers and upper managers need to support the concept fully in order to achieve success. Some suspicion may initially be felt as nursing roles change. The nurse manager may feel threatened by the introduction of another individual who is also managing care on the unit.

Before the advent of the prospective payment system, flex-time, increased severity levels, and technology, it was the nurse manager who carried out many of the role functions associated with managed care, such as facilitation and co-ordination of patient care services. As the nurse manager's role expanded and became more administrative, the nurse had less time to focus on managing the quality of care. Emphasize that the new concept will allow the nurse manager to concentrate more on administrative functions, which will in turn mean patients receive a higher quality of care. Reducing the sense of personal threat is essential to effecting a positive change.

STAFF INTEGRATION

If the nursing CEO was the one who initiated the change to case management, then the staff might already accept the change. If this is the case, then conversation with this group should concentrate on explaining the case management concept thoroughly and the changes it will bring.

The need to educate and fully enlist the support of the staff nurses cannot be emphasized enough. If the organization has decided to create the case manager position as a staff position, then staff nurses must be fully aware of the role. The job expectations of the case manager should be clear. If available, the job description should be distributed and reviewed. The role of the case manager in relation to other nursing positions should be made as clear as possible.

As with the introduction of any new position, there might be some initial role blending, role conflict, or both. This can be minimized through open discussion and ongoing review of the role after implementation. Nurses should anticipate that roles and responsibilities will evolve over time. The fluid nature of the position means it can be improved and enhanced as a part of the evaluation process.

The collaborative nature of the model means that all disciplines must support it. At the top of this list are the physicians. Getting the involvement of both medical physicians and surgeons will require varying techniques, with emphasis placed on the outcomes that are achievable for their patients. Rogers says: "It is important to use nurses well-known to the physicians who have a history of solid communication, mutual trust, clinical experience, and an overall positive experiential record. This serves to gain the initial support of physicians who might otherwise be resistant."*

For the surgeon who is reimbursed on a case basis, the incentive to discharge the patient more rapidly is a financial one because the discharge of one patient allows for the admission of the next. In addition, surgeons have traditionally treated patients in a protocoled manner. In this setting, the applicability of the case management approach is easily understood and appreciated. Because the surgical patient generally runs a predictable course of recovery, care can be planned in a very organized way. For this reason, surgeons will probably be those most receptive to implementation of the concept.

The medical physician, however, may pose a greater challenge. Currently, no financial incentives motivate these professionals to discharge patients more rapidly. Furthermore, it may be more difficult to predict the course of events for a particular medical diagnosis or condition.

---

*Rogers, M. (1992). Personal communication.

Incentives motivating the medical physician toward an appreciation of the case management approach will probably not be based on length-of-stay improvements. Emphasizing improved quality of care that will result may be one way to enlist physician support. Emphasis on the role of the case manager who, with the multidisciplinary action plan, can assure that the physician's best plan is initiated and followed may also help enlist support.

In some cases other initiatives may be useful. If the institution has several medical diagnoses whose lengths of stay are beyond state or federal averages, these should be targeted for initial intervention. In these cases, the chief physician may need to intervene. Essentially a practice guideline would be established that all physicians caring for a particular type of patient would be expected to follow. Whenever possible, active and positive participation is preferred.

Chart review and research are other techniques used to sell a treatment plan for a particular medical condition. Chart review often uncovers many ways for treating a medical problem. Each plan may not be equally effective, financially appropriate concerning resource use, or equally appropriate in terms of length of stay. By using chart review, inappropriate physician and nursing treatment interventions can be enhanced. The way other institutions treat particular types of problems can be used as a resource when determining the best possible treatment plan.

Standardized treatment plans are a great resource and asset for the resident or intern house staff. In addition, the case manager serves as a skilled resource for the new physician who is rotating through a particular nursing unit and is unfamiliar with the patient's present or past condition. In addition, the case manager helps the house officer elicit quick and accurate information. Ongoing dialogue between the two helps assure that the best plan will be implemented and carried out.

Case management will not be completely successful without the support and cooperation of ancillary departments. It is doubtful that an ancillary department will have an objection to the model although passive support is not enough to ensure success. To empower the case manager, a contact person in each department should be assigned to whom needs or concerns about patients can be referred.

Some areas will play a bigger part than others. For example, the radiology department plays a key role in some length-of-stay issues. Appropriate scheduling of tests in terms of order and timeliness is crucial to an early diagnosis and treatment. Appropriate preps also ensure that the patient's movement through the hospital is smooth.

Other ancillary departments, which play a key role in the case management model, are the admitting office, the DRG office, and the medical records department. Failure to obtain the support and commitment of these departments will result in difficulties during implementation and evaluation of the model.

Clearly other direct care providers must be fully supportive and committed for the model to be most effective. Key areas for such support include social work, physical therapy, and nutrition. The patient problem or surgery determines the areas most vital at any particular time, but certainly each department should be fully educated and agreeable before implementation.

Most ancillary departments appreciate the opportunity to work collaboratively with other disciplines. Nursing is not the only discipline plagued by frustration because of the divergent directions taken by each group of providers.

PLANNED CHANGE

A plan for implementation will provide the foundation for successful change. Each element outlined in this chapter should be evaluated and acted upon if appropriate for the institution. Planning for implementation should be carefully thought out and choreographed. The nine-step plan for implementation outlined in the box provides the foundation for the plan and identifies subsequent changes.

NINE-STEP PLAN FOR IMPLEMENTATION

- Define target patient populations.
- Match patient populations to nursing units.
- Determine design structure.
- Form multidisciplinary groups.
- Choose benchmarks.
- Collect preimplementation data.
- Provide advanced skills and knowledge.
- Implement model.
- Evaluate model.

This nine-step process provides a structure for planning any implementation program. Each element will be reviewed, and each aspect should be covered during the planning process. The ordering of each step may vary depending on the institution and certain steps may occur simultaneously.

Clearly the order is not as important as the actual carrying out of each step. This implementation process should be shared with everyone in the organization as the process is begun. The plan's steps for implementation, the ways in which those steps will be carried out, and the method of evaluation should be shared openly so that all those concerned have a chance to give input.

Because it will be advantageous to demonstrate some immediate success, selecting where to begin will be very important. A bad choice may mean failure or the cancellation of plans for adding units or teams to the model.

Target patient populations should be selected based on the following factors:

- Volume of discharges
- Variance from length-of-stay standards
- Variance from length-of-stay at similar institutions
- Feasibility of developing managed care plans
- Potential for control of resource consumption
- Opportunity for improvement in quality of care

If the organization's goal for implementation is to improve quality of care, this may be an additional factor taken into consideration during the selection process. This determination can be made through chart reviews of targeted populations.

Once the selection of patient populations has been made, these patients should be matched to appropriate nursing units. In some cases the type of patient group selected may not be found in one particular area of the hospital; therefore, a *non unit-based* case management team approach may be more appropriate.

In other cases, it will be possible to gather patients from a designated geographic area. The more homogeneous the patient population on a nursing unit is, the fewer the necessary resources will be in terms of physicians and managed care plans. This will result in a greater number of patients positively affected by the model.

Once the nursing unit, geographic area, or patient type has been selected, the design structure should be determined. If a *unit-based* model is being introduced, a determination must be made as to how many case managers will be on the unit. This decision will be based on the number of patient beds, the severity of the patients, the average length of stay, and the available resources. If only one position is available for conversion, this may be the deciding factor.

If a *non unit-based* case management model is being implemented, different factors will need to be taken into consideration. Most case management teams have members from several disciplines. Therefore this type of team may require a greater number of resources for implementation. A physician, nurse, social worker, and others need to be deployed. This may mean taking them away from other jobs or assignments, thereby requiring a greater financial commitment from the organization. The disciplines represented will depend on the particular clinical case type being followed by the team. For example, a diabetes team will clearly need a nutritionist and a social worker. Consultants with an affiliation to the team might include a podiatrist or an ophthalmologist.

In the *unit-based* model, the teams will have a fluid structure, and the members of the team will be constantly changing. The only constant member will be the unit-based case manager. The patient, physician, social worker, and so on, will change as the professionals assigned to the patient change. For each new patient, the case manager will need to gather a team, identify who is responsible for which aspects of the care plan, and ensure that everyone is working toward the same goals.

In the *non unit-based* case management model, the professional team members will remain constant, and the only changing member will be the patient. In this model, the team members and their respective roles are clearly defined up front, so there is no need to bring the group together.

As discussed in another chapter, choosing the outcome measures or benchmarks is a very important step. Selection of benchmarks must be done as early as possible and certainly before implementation. The method of evaluation will depend on the outcome measures chosen and the resources available for tracking the data.

Once the benchmarks have been selected, the method for data collection should be determined. The time frames should be documented in advance and the individuals responsible for the various elements should be identified.

It may be necessary and appropriate to enlist the help of employees from other departments who have access to certain pieces of data. For example, a representative from the DRG office or the medical records department might be assigned the responsibility of monitoring and tracking the length-of-stay data.

A representative from the quality improvement department might be recruited to track quality-of-care data on a quarterly basis. In some cases, it may even be possible to use students to assist with staff and patient questionnaires. A patient representative might be another good choice of someone to help with patient satisfaction questionnaires.

Regardless of the data being evaluated, baseline data sets must be established before education or implementation of the model. If the staff is being tested via questionnaires, those questionnaires must be distributed and returned before implementation. Some of the data will be retrospective; therefore the actual time when the data is pulled together will not be as important.

In Chapter 12, the elements of a good educational program are reviewed and discussed. It is critical that employees from all departments understand the general concepts of a case management system. To attain such understanding, an educational program may be offered, but the extent of such a program will vary depending on the resources available.

The case managers should be provided with as extensive a program as possible. It cannot be assumed that an employee comes to the position with the skills and knowledge necessary to carry out the role effectively. An investment and commitment from the organization for providing advanced skills and knowledge will help develop highly effective case managers. The need for education cannot be overemphasized.

In order to prevent contamination of subjects, educational preparation must follow any pre-implementation data collection. This maintains the integrity of the study sample.

IMPLEMENTING THE MODEL

Once all of the previous steps have been accomplished, the model can be effectively implemented. The date for beginning should be clearly communicated. The case management documentation system that has been selected may or may not be in place; although it is desirable, it is not essential. The case manager can begin changing the system immediately after entering the position. Having the case manager begin the changes might be the only practical way because other employees will not have the time or advanced skills necessary to make this change.

The question is often asked, "How do we begin?" The answer to this question is simple—*by beginning*. The transition phase, or the time between announced implementation and a full integration of the change, may be as long as a year or more. Therefore, after completing all pre-implementation steps, the case manager can smooth in the change gradually. It will take many months for all those involved to adjust to the system.

This time period will require communication with other members of the health care team, letting them know that the changeover has taken place and exactly what that means to them and to the organization. The more open and candid the communication, the more likely that the change will be accepted. The beginning is when many organizations falter, because they expect much of the change to have already been done. This expectation, however, is not practical. Everyone must understand in advance that the bulk of the changes will be phased in slowly.

PLANNING FOR EVALUATION

Evaluation of the model involves rigorous data collection and analysis. Unit Six will cover the evaluation process in detail. The time frames for analysis will be driven by the data elements themselves. It will be appropriate for some data, such as length of stay, to be collected and analyzed on a monthly basis. Other data, such as patient satisfaction, may only need to be tracked every 6 months. Annual tracking of staff satisfaction will be sufficient.

In addition to this formal data collection and analysis, an informal evaluation should be ongoing. Those responsible for the model should never forget to query practitioners who work within the model on a day-to-day basis at the patient bedside. Through discussions with the staff nurses and others, problem areas can be identified and corrective action taken. This ongoing dialogue may continue for one to two years while the change is being integrated. As the model expands, more and more employees will be affected. Barriers for successful integration will continue to appear as the model expands in sophistication and sphere of influence.

12

Education

CHAPTER OVERVIEW

Education is an essential element for successful implementation of a case management model. This chapter reviews the two types of curriculum required for implementation of a case management model. The first program, a general orientation to a case management model, is geared to a wide array of health care practitioners. The second program is a 3-day seminar designed to educate and train potential case managers. This chapter provides topical outlines and objectives for each program.

CURRICULUM DEVELOPMENT

Since case management's introduction in 1985, implementation has often called for elaborate planning, meetings, time, and commitment. What has been lacking to this point is a formal means of educating the staff nurses, case managers, and other personnel who might be interacting with the case manager.

Although case management theory has been introduced into some undergraduate as well as graduate curricula, those employees already in the health care field probably have not been introduced to the concepts through formal education. The length of the institution's educational program will depend on the time that can be donated to reallocating workers from their units to attend classroom instruction. For the most part, the concepts of case management are relatively new to most employees, so didactic teaching methods are important.

The amount of time set aside for instruction can range from 3 to 6 or more hours. However, the longer the program, the less likely it will be that employees from other disciplines will be able to be included. Although it is crucial that all staff nurses and ancillary nursing personnel attend these introductory sessions, it is also important for members of other disciplines to participate. The number of hours that these employees can be present in the program will depend on the staffing patterns of their departments. Although other disciplines may feel very committed to the case management model, they may not have the financial or personnnel resources available to allow workers to leave their jobs for more than one hour. For off-peak shifts, participation may be even less possible. It may be necessary to provide different programs of varying lengths to ensure that everyone can attend. It is the material that is important here, not the length of the program.

The topical outline for an introduction to a case management program should contain the following essential elements. Development of the curriculum should reflect all elements and characteristics of the case management process (Torres & Stanton, 1982). Other topics might be added depending on the needs of the organization. The more preparation and education provided to all members of the organization, the higher the chance is for success. Even those departments not directly involved with the program should be invited to attend. While not immediately obvious, areas such as the pharmacy or the radiology department will eventually be affected by a switch to case management. At the very least, all administrators and executive management should be encouraged to attend. Those involved in operations in the hospital can provide valuable insight into elements of the successful functioning of the model. Other departments—such as medicine, social work, quality assurance, utilization review, the patient representative department, nutrition, medical records, and admitting—are vital for the success of a case management model. Even though some individuals in these departments may be familiar with the case management concept, it is still important to educate them on how case management will be implemented in their organization. Such instruction will help prevent misunderstandings.

MULTIDISCIPLINARY EDUCATION

The contents of a program geared to a broad audience must be general enough to hold the attention of a wide range of health care providers, administrators, and operations personnel. This is no easy task. Specific examples of how case management might affect some of these workers will be helpful and should be included in the program.

It is vital to begin the presentation with an overview of case management. This overview should include the evolution of nursing delivery models. This information will provide the groundwork from which to start. Next, explain the relevance of case management in light of today's health care issues. Covering such topics will answer the "Why case management?" and "Why now?" questions. An understanding of the changes in health care reimbursement, the nursing shortage, changes in the current patient population, and other health care issues will help explain why case management is timely and essential for the continued success of most health care organizations. This framework for discussion will enable the audience to see that case management is not just a nursing project or a nursing problem. Not only does case management need them; they also need case management.

Empowering the Case Manager

Introduction of the case manager and introduction of the managed care plans are the two most essential changes to occur with the implementation of a case management model. Although many, more-subtle changes will occur, these are the two changes from which all the others will come.

The case manager must be empowered, and one technique for empowering is ensuring that everyone in the organization knows what a case manager does, and how the case manager fits into workers' daily routines. If a case manager calls to speak to the patient representative and the patient representative does not understand the case manager's role and function, then problems arise.

Topical Outline

A curriculum that addresses a wide audience can cover an array of relevant topics that are applicable to all employees (see Table 12-1). The following is a list of possible topics:
Define the concepts of case management.
Describe the role of the case manager.
Define the relationship between DRGs and case management.
Understand the use of the managed care plan.
Identify the case management outcomes for evaluation or research.
Defining the concepts of case management can be extensive or limited, depending on the audience. An overview should include discussion of previous nursing care delivery models, current health care crises, and health care reimbursement methods in reference to case management.

Discussion should include the evolution of the functional, team, and primary models and how these models relate to the case management model. After all, case management combines elements of team and primary nursing models.

Because the institutions may implement either a unit-based, free-floating or combined case management model, the subtle variations should be explored and discussed. This discussion should include the ways in which the various versions are structured, organized, and implemented.

Finally, a general overview of the expected outcomes of the case management model should be covered. The expected outcomes provide a relevant arena from which to set the case management goals for the organization as well as for the individual workers.

Role of the Case Manager

The role of the case manager must be included. During implementation, many false conceptions of the role develop, and this is usually caused by a lack of understanding. Professionals from other disciplines may draw their own conclusions as to what the case manager should or should not be doing. Although some role blending is necessary, education is the main way to avoid role confusion. (Kahn, Wolfe, Quinn, Snoek & Rosenthal, 1964).

The case manager job description should be distributed during the educational sessions, or at the very least, it should be reviewed. This is the first step in distinguishing the roles and responsibilities of the case manager. Such steps will help ensure that other disciplines will respect the boundaries of the case manager's job description, and will not expect the manager to function beyond it. It is possible that some workers may expect case managers to be less influential than

Table 12-1   General orientation program content outline

Objectives	Content

Define the concepts of case management.	Overview
	    Managed care vs. case management
	    Evolution of nursing delivery models

Describe the role of the case manager.	Review
	    Job description
	    Job responsibilities
	    Daily operations
	    Relationship to other disciplines

Explain the relationship between DRGs and case management; explain the use of managed care plans.	DRGs
	    Definition/changes in reimbursement
	    Relationship and link to case management
	    Use of managed care plans and their relationship to DRGs

Identify the case management outcomes for research.	Research outcomes
	    Improved registered nurse satisfaction
	    Decreased burnout
	    Decreased length of stay
	    Improved patient satisfaction
	    Improved quality of care

outlined in their job descriptions. Others may expect duties beyond the scope of their job descriptions. A clear description of the role set forth in the beginning will help minimize misunderstandings (O'Malley, 1988).

A clear way in which to define and illustrate the job functions of the case manager is through a description of daily operations, as well as a description of what the case manager's typical day might be like. It is not uncommon to be asked, *What exactly does a case manager do?* Like many jobs of this nature, the specific tasks are often invisible or intangible or both. Once again, the theoretic framework of the model and the expected outcomes should be emphasized.

Review of the Health Care Reimbursement System

Managed care's basic premise is based on achieving expected outcomes of care within appropriate time frames. A portion of the curriculum should be devoted to reviewing the present health care reimbursement system. It is around this system that much of case management lies (Hartley, 1986). Other points to be covered should include how DRGs work, and how these predetermined lengths of stay determine reimbursement rates.

DRGs are used in case management to help determine the number of days on which to base managed care plans. This relationship should be defined in detail. Other uses of the managed care plans should also be reviewed, including the ways in which they are used to maintain quality in an accelerated health care system. The links between quality and cost in a case management environment should be reviewed.

Projected Outcomes

The projected outcomes of the model can be covered next. The general goals of any case management model and the specific goals of the organization should be covered. This section will include topics, such as improved quality of care, improved caregiver satisfaction, improved patient satisfaction, decreased length of stay, and decreased resource utilization.

Once again, the length and detail of this program must be determined by the audience and the amount of time that can be allotted by the various departments.

CASE MANAGER EDUCATION

Several days should be devoted to educating the case managers. It cannot be assumed that nurses newly promoted to the role of case manager can function without training. Individual organizations will need to decide the person(s) best qualified to provide this education. In some cases, outside consultants or experts in the field may be needed to provide this service.

In a 3-day program, two of the days should be devoted to case management concepts, and one day should be devoted to leadership/management training. It will be likely that nurses promoted to case management roles will have had no experience in either managing or case management.

Day One

The differences between leadership and management should be explained during the first day (see Table 12-2). Functioning as a case manager will require the use of both roles (Holle & Blatchley, 1987).

Some suggested topics to be covered might include the qualities of a leader, the correlation between administration style and the nursing process, contingency management theory, and accountability versus responsibility. While the case manager role is not identifiable as a management position in the traditional sense, it is essential that the case manager understands these concepts and will be able to use them to effect the changes necessary for achieving excellent outcomes.

The case manager must be empowered. A portion of this perceived empowerment must be inherent in the individual assuming the role (Bennis & Nanus, 1985). A working knowledge of the theories of power and their relationship to the role of the case manager should be included in the curriculum. Case managers should understand that their personal power sources are as related to their personal style as those found in the job description. Strategies for obtaining as well as using power should be reviewed. A positive use of power will enhance self-esteem and bring more effectiveness to the role.

Implementation of a case management model involves subtle as well as obvious changes. It has been said that change is painful but just how painful depends on the level of organizational support as well as individual support. Understanding the stages and processes of change can help decrease the difficulties associated with changes. Whether the organization is large or small, complex or simple,

Table 12-2   Case manager education day one content outline

Objectives	Content

Define leadership vs. management.	Leadership vs. management
	    Definitions of leadership and management
	    Qualities of a leader
	    Difference between administrative process and nursing process
	    Contingency management (situational management)
	    Accountability vs. responsibility

Describe power and its uses for a case manager.	Definition of power
	    Definition of power
	    Five sources of power
	    Constructive and destructive uses of power
	    Strategies to obtain power

Identify the change process.	Change theory
	    Three types of change
	        Technical
	        Structural
	        People-oriented
	    Lewin's Phases of Change
	        Freezing
	        Moving
	        Exploring
	        Refreezing
	        Implementation
	    Effecting positive change in management
	    Ten conditions that make change acceptable
	    Approaches to decreasing resistance to change

Relate the concepts of power and change.	Relationship between power and change
	    Empowerment
	    Change = empowerment: empowerment = change

Demonstrate effective communication techniques.	Communication
	    Do's and don'ts of effective communication
	    Active listening
	    Assertive vs. aggressive behavior
	    Conflict
	        Source
	        Resolutions
	    Problem-solving strategies

Describe the process of patient education.	Patient education
	    Adult learning principles
	    Strategies for effective teaching and learning

State the legal rights of patients.	Legal rights of patients
	    Patient bill of rights
	    Health care proxy
	    Living will
	    Do-not-resuscitate (DNR) laws

Implement discharge planning process.	Discharge planning
	    Collaborative process
	    Assessment and planning
	    Referrals to provide continuity of care

change is never easy and seldom goes smoothly. If the case manager understands this in advance, any difficulties can be lessened along with the possible ambiguities experienced by other workers with whom the manager comes in contact.

The specific theory of change used by the instructor is not as important as conveying the message that the conversion to case management will be bumpy, and that some days will not be productive or fulfilling. Nevertheless, the case manager should understand the techniques for effecting positive change and the conditions that make change more acceptable.

Implementation will always involve some resistance. A portion of the organization will accept the change immediately, some will be resistant, and others will remain in the middle of the road reserving their judgments until they see the model in action for themselves. It will be impossible to win everyone over, and the case manager should understand this. Approaches to reducing resistance to change might be employed to help make the transition as smooth as possible.

Power and change are interrelated concepts. An empowered individual is in a better position to effect change. At the same time, the more change effected, the more empowered the individual becomes.

The effectiveness of any leader or manager is dependent upon the styles of communication used. A substantial portion of the curriculum should be devoted to teaching effective communication techniques. One topic that can make a difference in the successful integration of the case manager role is the use of proper verbal and nonverbal communication styles, as well as proper techniques for listening. Active listening can result in positive communication interactions.

Integrated in this should also be the technique for assertive communication versus the aggressive communication style, which has been shown to be less effective.

Finally, the case manager should be aware of the various sources of conflict that may come about as a result of the intregration of this role, and the problem-solving strategies that should be used for resolving conflict.

Patient education is an integral part of the case manager role. It is one of the three main role functions. Therefore the principles of adult learning and strategies for effective teaching and learning should be included in the curriculum. Effective inpatient teaching is an aid to successful recovery at home.

The case manager must serve as a patient advocate as she interacts on the patient's behalf with other departments and disciplines. This advocacy role is possibly more important than it has ever been. The curriculum should include a discussion of DNR (Do Not Resuscitate) laws, living wills, and health care proxy laws. A lecturer with expertise in these areas should be recruited.

A portion of the curriculum should cover discharge planning, with an emphasis on collaboration. The role of the social worker is very important in the discharge planning process, and a social worker should be enlisted to provide insights on how case manager and social worker roles should work together. Many disciplines share the responsibility of assessing and planning for discharge. Reaching out to the community is part of the discharge planning process. As much as possible, the case manager should be made aware of the various community resources available for varying patient problems. Some of these referral sources will come to the case manager's attention once the manager begins working in the role; nevertheless, an overview of some of the resources available should be covered.

Day Two

The second day (see Table 12-3) should provide an overview and definition of case management. The relationship between cost and quality should be reviewed as they relate to case management along with the goals of a case management model. Also included in an overview should be an in-depth historical perspective of the evolution of nursing care delivery models. This will help to put today's case management model in perspective and give it relevance.

Case management is important as it relates to the current health care environment. There are numerous relevant health care crises, but some of the top ones might include the current nursing shortage, changes in health care reimbursement as related to the prospective payment system, an aging patient population, the AIDS epidemic, and increased technology in health care. Case management has evolved out of the current crises. Presenting case management from its historical perspective will lend relevance to the model.

The prospective payment system needs to be covered in detail because it is this system of predetermined lengths of stay as related to the DRG system that has been one of the reasons the concept of case management evolved. The system should be covered in its entirety. Differences between what the state calls an acceptable length of stay and what the federal government calls acceptable should be provided. The case manager must understand the reimbursement system completely and must be fluent with the terms related to it. Guest lecturers who have expertise in this area or others should be invited to speak whenever possible.

The role functions and responsibilities of the case manager should be covered, with a review of the case manager job description. The collaborative relationship between the case manager and all other disciplines should be emphasized. The specific responsibilities of the case manager can be covered during this time. These responsibilities would include education, discharge planning, and facilitation of the patient through the system.

The managed care plan can be reviewed for form, content, and purpose. Possible topics to be covered when discussing the managed care plans might include the following: design, documentation, relationship to length of stay, use as a collaborative tool, and quality-of-care monitoring. The managed care plans should be reviewed in detail, as they are one of the more visible and tangible changes in case management. Methods for writing the managed care plan should be reviewed. Included in this portion of the education should be the ways in which a managed care plan can be used to track variances in care and quality data. Tracking and trending for selected patient problems or entire disease entities can be followed concurrently or retrospectively through the managed care format.

Table 12-3   Case manager education day two content outline

Objectives	Content

Define the concepts of case management.	Overview of case management
	    Definition
	    Nine steps to case management
	    Goals of case management
	    Expected outcomes of case management

Identify issues affecting health care delivery in the 1990s.	Health care crisis
	    Nursing shortage
	    Changes in reimbursement
	    Aging population
	    AIDS epidemic
	    Increased technology

Explain the DRG reimbursement system.	Fiscal issues facing nursing
	    DRGs
	    Length of stay

State the role of case manager and other members of the health care team.	Professional image
	    Case manager job description
	    Collaborative roles
	        Nursing
	        Physicians
	        Social work

Define managed care plans.	Managed care plans
	    Design
	    Documentation
	    Relationship to length of stay
	    Collaborative tool
	    Education
	    Quality of care

Document accurately the changes in case management using the managed care plan.	Changes
	    Length of stay
	    Patient/practitioner variances
	    Quality of care

Identify appropriate strategies for measuring, evaluating and assessing outcomes.	Quality assurance documentation
	    Problem-solving techniques
	    Tracking and trending: selection of population source data
	    Development of monitoring tool
	    Analysis of data
	    Evaluation and followup

Day Three

The third day (see Table 12-4) should include a review of the roles and functions of the case manager. A "train the trainer" approach is useful during this portion of the curriculum. If someone already in the role of case manager is available, it is much more worthwhile for the new case manager to hear exactly how the role is carried out from someone who is already functioning in the role. A thorough review of how the case manager should collect data on patients should be provided. These data provide a framework for the case manager to track the patients while in the hospital and after discharge. Although each case

Table 12-4   Case manager education day three content outline

Objectives	Content
Identify role of case manager.	Video tape
Complete the managed care plan.	Review plans, practice writing
Discuss variance analysis.	How to determine and analyze variances
Discuss differentiated practice.	Discuss the relationship of differentiated practice and case management
Role play.	Introduction of patient/physician/RN/ other disciplines

manager will individualize the data collection process, some standard methods can be reviewed. In addition, walking the case manager through the day is also helpful.

A workshop dedicated to managed care plan writing is a must for the third day. Each case manager should be given the opportunity to write a managed care plan from beginning to end. Going through the process step by step helps identify areas of confusion or uncertainty.

Variance analysis is one of the unique opportunities provided by a case management model. By retrospectively analyzing what did or did not happen and looking for patterns as well as causes of the variances, then justification for changes in care can be made (Blaney & Hobson, 1988). The case manager should be well-versed in this process. In addition to providing the rationale for changes in care plans, variance analysis will allow for future upgrading of the quality of care. It is much easier to track clinical outcomes using the variance analysis format.

Many case management programs use some differentiated practice methods. Differentiated practice calls for the assignment of personnel based on employee level of education, experience, and expertise (AHA, 1990). An effective case management program should fold in a differentiated practice system so that optimal use can be made of the nurse's experience and education. One part of case management training should cover the levels of education for nurses and should include a discussion of the strengths and weaknesses associated with each of these education levels.

One period of the curriculum should be devoted to role-playing. Such role-playing will help case managers by walking them through some of the situations they will encounter. One of the hardest areas for some new case managers is explaining to patients, physicians, and others exactly what the case manager role is about. Giving out business cards to patients is equally difficult because the case managers are not familiar with such formalities. Practice with the card can address and solve these problems. This may seem rudimentary, but it is crucial that the case manager feel at ease with these tasks.

Role-playing can also be used to practice ways of confronting and resolving conflicts that arise during the change process.

REFERENCES

American Hospital Association (1990). *Current issues and perspective on differentiated practice.* Chicago: American Organization of Nurse Executives.

Bennis, W., & Nanus, B. (1985). *Leaders.* New York: Harper & Row.

Blaney, D.R., & Hobson, C.J. (1988). *Cost-effective nursing practice: Guidelines for nurse managers.* New York: J.B. Lippincott Company.

Hartley, S. (1986). Effects of prospective pricing on nursing. *Nursing Economics, 4*(1), 16-18.

Holle, M.L., & Blatchley, M.E. (1987). *Introduction to leadership and management in nursing.* Boston: Jones & Bartlett.

Kahn, R.L., Wolfe, D.M., Quinn, R.P., Snoek, J.D., & Rosenthal, R.A. (1964). *Organizational stress: Studies in role conflict and ambiguity.* New York: Wiley.

O'Malley, J. (1988). Nursing care management, part II: Dimensions of the nurse case manager role. *Aspen's Advisor for Nurse Executives, 3*(7), 8-9.

Torres, G., & Stanton, M. (1982). *Curriculum process in nursing: A guide to curriculum development,* Englewood Cliffs, N.J.: Prentice-Hall.

Zander, K. (1992 Fall). Quantifying, managing, and improving quality. Part III. Using variance concurrently. *The New Definition, 7*(4), 1-4.

IMPLEMENTATION

13

The Cast of Characters

CHAPTER OVERVIEW

Primary nursing models no longer meet the changing needs of either the hospital environment or the patients. In this chapter the multidisciplinary approach is discussed in terms of its relative value to the case management model. Both this approach and case management in general are presented in response to an increasingly complex health care environment. How to form teams and how to gain the support and trust of colleagues are two of the topics discussed.

GETTING OUT OF THE PARALLEL PLAY SYNDROME

Those who began their nursing careers in the, 1970s were trained and educated to function as independent and professional nurses. With the advent of the primary nursing model, *professional* meant doing everything oneself (Bakke, 1974). The team spirit and sense of esprit de corps were lost in the fight to prove nursing a worthy profession. In the attempt to show just how important nursing was to the patient, other disciplines, which also provided unique and necessary services, were neglected.

Perhaps nursing had to go through this process. Perhaps it was necessary as part of the profession's evolutionary growth. Because nursing was so used to being viewed as a second-class profession, nurses were riding high on the conviction that they could do it all and do it all well.

Out of this generation of parallel play came terms such as *burnout, fatigue syndrome,* and *fragmented care.* Under the primary nursing model, it was expected that the nurse would meet all of the patient's needs, from the bed bath to the discharge plan. With the nursing shortage that began in 1985 and the prospective payment system that resulted in shortened lengths of stay, nurses found it almost impossible to function under the primary nursing system.

Increased complexity and technology required that registered nurses become experts in a narrower range of tasks, which meant that other tasks had to be relinquished or returned to the other disciplines. Nursing care had to become more specialized as it responded to changing patient needs both in the hospital and after discharge.

103

Because the hospital stay was shortened by the prospective payment system, the phrase "discharge them quicker, but sicker" was being quoted by both health care practitioners and patients. Members of the public were losing confidence in the health care system because they felt rushed through the process by the insurers as well as the health care providers who now had to keep the hospital stay as short as possible.

Flexible time (flex-time) measures, which were designed to attract more people to the profession and to retain those already in the workforce, contributed to fragmented nursing care. Fragmentation was chiefly an outcome of these measures, which resulted in the advent of 10- and 12-hour shifts. Flex-time was very attractive to employees because it allowed them to have long blocks of time off to spend with their families and to continue their education.

Unfortunately, these long blocks of time created a tremendous gap in patient care. Trying to be all things to the patient for 12 hours and then not being present for 3 days was meeting the worker's needs at the patient's expense. The situation was compounded by the accelerated hospital stay. It was conceivable that patients might see a different nurse during each day of an average 4-day hospital stay. Patients complained that no one knew them or their needs, and they were unable to develop professional relationships with any of their nurses. These patients felt that no one practitioner was responsible for their care. Nursing appeared to have failed because accountability for patient care had been lost.

Although nursing departments across the country tried to keep functioning in primary nursing systems, the new environment made it impossible to do so. Primary nursing had been founded on the notion that the registered professional nurse would be responsible for all aspects of the patient's care from admission to discharge. This became unattainable with the introduction of the flex-time system. Although nurses were theoretically responsible, extended absences from the unit prevented a true continuation of their relationship with the patient or the other members of the health care team.

In addition to this, patient assignments continued, in many instances, to remain geographic, with each nurse on the shift assigned a particular geographic part of the nursing unit. If the patient was moved to some other area of the unit, it was likely that the primary nurse would no longer be caring for that patient. Such changes meant care had become extremely fragmented.

At the same time, the role of the head nurse or nurse manager was moving away from the bedside. More and more administrative responsibility was given to these middle managers as upper management positions were eliminated. In the past the nurse manager had been able to clinically monitor all the patients on the floor and still carry out managerial responsibilities. As the administrative duties increased, this became more difficult to accomplish. In addition, the average length of stay was dramatically shortened so that patients were admitted and discharged from the unit faster than they could be followed by a busy manager with other responsibilities.

THE EFFECTS OF A CHANGING ENVIRONMENT

It was during the 1970s that nurses and other health care providers first began to complain of stress-related problems such as chronic fatigue and burnout. In 1974, a psychologist named Freudenberger coined the clinical term *burnout* in the literature. Burnout was described as the degeneration of a once highly productive individual into a negative, exhausted one. It was seen as a direct response to work stress when the worker no longer had the resources available to deal with other people's emotional, psychologic, and physical problems.

Burnout follows a particular pattern that generally begins with feelings of emotional exhaustion. Such exhaustion is a result of being emotionally overextended and exhausted by one's work with others (Maslach, 1976, 1978, 1982). This exhaustion is followed by feelings of depersonalization, which have been described as negative, unfeeling, and impersonal responses toward the recipients of one's care (Maslach, 1976, 1978, 1982). As the syndrome becomes more severe, the worker may describe feelings of reduced personal accomplishment. Personal accomplishment is characterized by feelings of competence and successful achievement in one's work with people (Maslach, 1976, 1978, 1982).

By placing registered nurses in a position that required them to be all things to the patient, the nurses experienced an incredible amount of on-the-job stress. Role overload was yet another outcome of work stress that was identified in some nurses (Cesta, 1989). Role overload is characterized by workers' subjective feelings of being unable to complete their work because of inadequate personal or environmental resources (French & Caplan, 1972; Hardy, 1976; Ritzer, 1977). These feelings have been reported to be particularly high in nurses who are in their first 2 years of employment (Cesta, 1989; Das, 1981; Maslach, 1982).

When role overload combined with feelings of burnout, the nurse's ability to deal with work began to change and gradually diminished (Cesta, 1989).

Nurses began to adjust the primary nursing system in an attempt to address changes in the health care arena. This new system eventually became known as *modified primary,* and retained the theory that the nurse was accountable for all aspects of care. However, this did not mean that the nurse retained responsibility for the patient from admission to discharge. Primary nursing responsibilities were applicable only to the day the nurse worked.

Once these modifications were made in the primary model, the stage was set for the development of a more appropriate model that addressed all of the above issues (Loveridge, Cummings, and O'Malley, 1988).

Nursing responded to the changes in health care by looking for an alternative patient care delivery model. The alternative was a model that combined elements of team and primary nursing (Zander, 1985). There was really nothing new or revolutionary about the case management model for nursing care delivery. The basic premise of the model was a team or collaborative approach that allowed the case manager to function as the evaluator and coordinator of care or facilitator of the team. This new role was similar to that of the primary nurse, except that the case manager was now removed from direct patient care responsibility.

With the addition of this role, nursing moved away from attempting to be all things to the patient. Members of the profession began to admit that they could not do all things equally well, that other members of the team were needed to provide their particular areas of expertise.

Nursing was finally getting out of the parallel play syndrome and was moving toward a more dynamic and interactive modality.

FORMATION OF THE COLLABORATIVE PRACTICE GROUPS

It is perhaps easier now for nurses to reintroduce themselves to the team approach. Although social workers and physicians had functioned that way for years, nurses had been struggling to achieve independence and autonomy. Nurses now feel more confident and ready to join the team after gaining prestige among other health care providers (Farley & Stoner, 1989).

Institutions implementing case management models for the first time must explain to team members why nurses are returning to the team approach. At first, this reintroduction of the team approach may be observed with some suspicion and doubt. Without making the intentions of the team clear it will be impossible to institute collaborative practice groups.

Many physicians and other health care providers may have preconceived ideas about case management. Some of these ideas may stem from their familiarity with managed care systems that have been introduced in HMOs. Generally, these managed care systems are seen as negative by many other health care providers. They are seen as just one more way for their practices to be regulated and controlled and their services to be rationed (Schwartz & Mendelson, 1992).

Collaborative practice groups cannot be formed until all members adopt the model as their own and see its benefit for both themselves and for the patient. It should be emphasized that case management is not just a nursing care model, but a way for all the disciplines to form plans of care that avoid duplication of effort, unnecessary tests and procedures, or misuse of resources.

Each discipline involved in patient care activities develops a plan that meets the objectives for that discipline as they relate to the patient. Case management provides, for the first time, the opportunity for all the disciplines to come together in an effort to use each other's expertise for maximum benefit to the patient.

Cast of Characters

Who then, comprise the cast of characters, and how do they come together as a group? Formation of these inter-disciplinary groups is one of the first steps for implementation, and it must take place before any real clinical changes can occur.

In a unit-based case management approach, the members of the group will be dependent upon the types of managed care plans being developed. At the least each group should consist of the following members from their respective disciplines: nursing, medicine, social work, and nutrition. People from these areas make up the core of any group, and each one provides input related to the clinical objectives of that member's discipline. Of course, the central figures in any such team are the patient and family.

Other members are added as they relate to the particular diagnosis or procedure planned. Other disciplines that might be included are physical therapy, respiratory therapy, psychiatry, and others as needed.

In some cases, the groups may have already been formed as part of the implementation of a non unit-based case management approach. In this approach, groups are formed around a particular diagnosis and all members of the team are experts in that clinical area.

For example, a team might be formed to manage diabetic patients throughout the hospital. A diabetes case management team is often headed by a diabetologist and a nurse case manager who provide the leadership to direct the other members of the team. A cardiac case management team might be headed by a cardiologist and a cardiac nurse case manager. The members of a case management team follow the patients' cases regardless of where they might be within the hospital. Therefore the team remains constant while the patients and their locations change.

Because the case management team is developed before the arrival of the patient, these groups have already determined protocols and care methods for their specific types of patients. It is not necessary for the case manager to identify the members of the team at the time of the patient's admission to the hospital, because the team is already in place.

However, in the unit-based case management model, the members of the team are dependent on the patient problem. These teams are fluid and constantly changing.

After admission, the attending physician, patient care manager, social worker, nutritionist, and others are identified, after which time the specific plan of care for the patient is formalized.

The use of internal techniques and relationships should not be underestimated in the formation of the multidisciplinary groups. If a nonthreatening, informal relationship has been developed first, it will be much easier to obtain the cooperation of some professionals. Inviting key players to lunch, meeting in the library, or just chatting on the unit can do much to gain trust and respect.

There may be occasions when a member of another discipline who is in a position of authority may be needed to intervene on the part of the case manager to obtain concurrence for collaborative practice. For example, some physicians admit large numbers of patients to the hospital every year and are therefore considered to carry a great deal of power and independence in their everyday practice within the hospital. These individuals may not immediately see the advantage of joining a multidisciplinary team effort, because it may not appear to benefit them, or they may view the effort to form teams as an attempt to control their practices. In a case like this, it may be necessary to have a physician administrator intervene on the behalf of the case management team. Usually, once the benefits are presented to the physicians, they give their support. Also, they may need to get their superiors consent to participate.

Another technique to gain the support of some of the more resistant professionals is to begin working first with those who have already agreed to the model. It is sometimes more effective to begin with these individuals than try to convert the resisters right away. Perhaps, when success is proved with those who have been immediately receptive, the others will eventually give their support. Once again, support may be dependent on people's perceptions of what the model can do for them. There will always be a certain percentage of players who will sit on the fence, waiting to see if implementation succeeds or fails. Once success is evident, they will then cross over to the case manager's side.

In both the unit- and non unit-based case management approach, the team becomes the focal point for care delivery, with each member lending information from a specific area of expertise. Most institutions rely on the case manager to be responsible for smooth operation and communication among team members. However, in some instances, social workers or physicians have been used to coordinate communication. Nurses function well in this role because they are educated to take a holistic approach to care delivery and because they are the ones who get involved in all aspects of the patient's care.

For example, it is less likely that a social worker will have the clinical skills that a registered nurse has but most registered nurses have the basic skills required to provide discharge planning and referral services to patients after discharge. At the very least, the case manager should be able to work the system to the patient's advantage, knowing which members to call when appropriate. An advanced understanding of the patient's medical and nursing needs helps to make this assessment complete. The case manager can then refer the problem to the appropriate practitioner.

In the unit-based approach, it may be difficult or impossible for the complete team to meet at one time. Once again, case managers fill this gap. They provide the thread that holds all the members together. In this sense, the case managers must have excellent and accurate skills of communication. The information they translate between team members and to patients and families must be accurate and concise. Otherwise, the thread is broken and the team falls apart.

The team should be assembled as a group whenever possible. Dialogue and opinion can thus be shared face-to-face. It is often during meetings of this type that difficult patient problems are resolved.

The case manager may spend a good deal of time during the beginning of implementation trying to ensure that the team becomes a reality and remains on target to provide the best possible care for the patient.

The case manager role consists of three dimensions (Tahan, 1992). The first dimension is the clinical role, which requires collaboration with the interdisciplinary team and involves the development of protocols that list the key tasks or events that must be accomplished for handling patient problems. Case managers use these protocols to direct, monitor, and evaluate patient treatment and the outcomes or responses to treatment (Thompson, Caddick, Mathie, Newlon & Abraham, 1991; Zander, 1988).

Case managers identify variances from the standard protocols and work with other health care team members to analyze and deal with these variances of care (Ethridge & Lamb, 1989; O'Malley, 1988b).

The second dimension is that of the managerial role, which refers to the case managers responsibility for coordinating the care of patients during the course of hospitalization (Ethridge & Lamb, 1989; Kruger, 1989; O'Malley, 1988a; Zander, 1988). The case manager manages care by planning the nursing treatment modalities and interventions necessary for meeting the needs of the patient and the family. Goals of treatment are set at admission, and length of stay is determined as it relates to the DRG. The discharge plan is formed as early in the hospital stay as possible (O'Malley, 1988b).

Case managers also guide the activities, nursing treatments, and interventions of other nursing staff members (Ethridge & Lamb, 1989; Kruger, 1989). They continuously evaluate the quality of care provided and outcomes of treatments and services to prevent misuse of resources (O'Malley, 1988a).

One of the informal responsibilities of the case manager is that of teacher and mentor (Cronin & Maklebust, 1989; Kruger, 1989). The case manager assesses staff development needs, especially among the less experienced practitioners, and refers them to the appropriate person or resource (Leclair, 1991). As part of the teaching responsibilities of the role, case managers conduct patient and family teaching sessions during the hospitalization period (Cronin & Maklebust, 1989; Zander, 1988).

The third dimension of the case manager role involves financial aspects. In collaboration with the physician and other health care members, case managers activate a caregiving process for each patient and use a case management plan, which is a generic tool for managing care and keeping it consistent with the predetermined financial outcomes for a defined case type (O'Malley, 1988b; Zander, 1988). The use of such clinical treatment standards helps ensure that patients do not receive inadequate care because of cost containment measures (Collard, Bergman & Henderson, 1990).

Case managers access information related to DRGs, the cost of each diagnosis, the allocated length of stay, and the treatments and procedures generally used for each diagnosis. They use this information to review resources and evaluate the efficiency of care related to the diagnosis (Cronin & Maklebust, 1989). The case manager has a great influence on the quality and price of care by helping to determine in a timely manner the most pertinent treatment for the patient (Henderson & Collard, 1988). Case managers also assess variances for each DRG and act immediately to control these variances to contain costs (Crawford, 1991). They assure consistency, continuity, and coordination of care to control for duplication and fragmentation in health care delivery, which results in better resource allocation and further cost containment (Henderson & Collard, 1988; O'Malley, 1988a).

To be effective, case managers must access information on case mix index, cost of resources, and consumption, and must be familiar with the prospective payment system and current third-party reimbursement procedures (Ethridge & Lamb, 1989; O'Malley, 1988b).

Case managers work closely with the utilization review department in identifying long-stay patients and planning with that department to control and prevent inappropriate hospital stays (Cronin & Maklebust, 1989).

REFERENCES

Bakke, K. (1974). Primary nursing: Perceptions of a staff nurse. *American Journal of Nursing, 74* (8), 1432-1434.

Cesta, T.G. (1989). "The Relationship of Role Overload and Burnout to Coping Process in Registered Professional Staff Nurses Newly Employed in a Hospital Setting." Doctoral Dissertation. University Microfilms, Inc., Publication Number: 9016399.

Collard, A.F., Bergman, A., & Henderson, M. (1990). Two approaches to measuring quality in medical case management programs. *Quality Review Bulletin, 3-8.*

Crawford, J. (1991). Managed care consultant: The "House supervisor" alternative. *Nursing Management, 22 (5),* 75-78.

Cronin, C.J., & Maklebust, J. (1989). Case-managed care: Capitalizing on the CNS. *Nursing Management, 20 (3),* 38-47.

Das, E.B.L. (1981). Contributing factors to burnout in the nursing environment (Doctoral dissertation, Texas Woman's University, 1981). *Dissertation Abstracts International, 42,* 04B.

Ethridge, P., & Lamb, G. (1989). Professional nursing case management improves quality, access and costs. *Nursing Management, 20 (3),* 30-35.

Farley, M.J., & Stoner, M.H. (1989). The nurse executive and interdisciplinary team building. *Nursing Administration Quarterly,* 24-29.

French, J.R.P., & Caplan, R.D. (1972). Organizational stress and individual strain. In A.J. Morrow (Ed.), *The failure of success* (pp. 30-66). New York: AMACOM.

Freudenberger, H.J. (1974). Staff burn-out. *Journal of Social Issues, 30,* 159-165.

Hardy, M.E. (1976). Role problems, role strain, job satisfaction, and nursing care. Paper presented at the annual meeting of the American Sociological Association, New York, August, 1976.

Henderson, M.G., & Collard, A. (1988). Measuring quality in medical case management programs. *Quality Review Bulletin,* 33-39.

Kruger, N.R. (1989). Case Management: Is it a delivery system for my organization? *Aspen's Advisor for Nurse Executives, 4 (10),* 4-6.

Leclair, C. (1991). Introducing and accounting for RN case management. *Nursing Management, 22 (3),* 44-49.

Loveridge, C.E., Cummings, S.H., & O'Malley, J. (1988). Developing case management in a primary nursing system. *Journal of Nursing Administration, 18 (10),* 36-39.

Maslach, C. (1976). Burned-out. *Human Behavior, 5,* 17-21.

Maslach, C. (1978). Job burn-out: How people cope. *Public Welfare, 36,* 56-58.

Maslach, C. (1982). *Burnout. The cost of caring.* Englewood Cliffs, N.J.: Prentice-Hall.

O'Malley, J. (1988a). Nursing case management, part I: Why look at a different model for nursing care delivery? *Aspen's Advisor for Nurse Executives, 3 (5),* 5-6.

O'Malley, J. (1988b). Nursing case management, part II: Dimensions of the nurse case manager role. *Aspen's Advisor for Nurse Executives, 3 (6),* 7.

Ritzer, G. (1977). *Working.* Englewood Cliffs, N.J.: Prentice-Hall.

Schwartz, W., & Mendelson, D. (1992 Summer). Why managed care cannot contain hospital cost without. *Health Affairs* 100-107.

Tahan, H. (1992). *The role of the case manager.* Manuscript submitted for publication.

Thompson, K.S., Caddick, K., Mathie, J., Newlon, B., & Abraham, T. (1991). Building a critical path for ventilator dependency. *American Journal of Nursing,* 28-31.

Zander, K. (1992 Fall). Quantifying, managing, and improving quality. Part III. Using variance concurrently. *The New Definition* 7(4):1-4.

Zander, K. (1985). Second generation primary nursing: A new agenda. *Journal of Nursing Administration, 15 (3),* 18-24.

Zander, K. (1988). Managed care within acute care settings: design and implementation via nursing case management. *Health Care Supervisor. 6 (2),* 27-43.

14

Variations Within Clinical Settings

CHAPTER OVERVIEW

Case management models provide an opportunity for health care institutions to provide quality, cost-effective services, regardless of the type of setting or financial resources. The model is flexible and can be adapted to meet the needs of both clinical and institutional settings.

This chapter describes the ways in which the case management model can be adapted to a variety of clinical settings, including medicine, surgery, critical care, nursing homes, and clinics. The way a case management model is used depends on the goals of the organization using it. The chapter also discusses the challenge facing case management in linking the inpatient and outpatient settings.

FLEXIBILITY OF CASE MANAGEMENT

One of the things that makes case management models particularly appealing is that the structure is extremely flexible. A case management design can be modified to fit the needs and budgets of any clinical setting. Because the primary goals of case management are to reduce costs while maintaining quality, the model can, in many circumstances, be implemented for a minimal cost (Ethridge & Lamb, 1989).

There are probably as many variations on the case management theme as there are nursing units in the United States. There is no right or wrong way to design a case management unit. The design is not as important as the roles and functions of the unit's members. Each person's functions are what make the model unique, not the number of workers involved.* Today's health care environment calls for flexibility and creativity, and the institutions that display these features will probably be the most successful ones over the next 10 years (Armstrong & Stetler, 1991).

For an institution implementing case management for the first time, the exact design structure for the units will be determined based on an array of factors.

---

*This is because the team becomes greater as a whole, than when each member functions independently.

Choosing the first units to participate is an important decision. If the first units are successful, the institution will be more likely to support continued implementation. On the other hand, if the first units are less than successful, the leaders of the organization may not be willing to allow the implementation process to continue. Therefore, the first units should be chosen carefully.

The units selected for initial implementation should have the following characteristics:

- Homogeneous patient population
- High volume case types
- Potential for improvement in length of stay
- A committed nurse manager
- A receptive physician group
- An interested nursing staff
- An open FTE position

Of course, it may not be possible to obtain each of these elements on every nursing unit. Finding a unit with as many of these factors as possible will help ensure a positive transition to a case management model.

A homogeneous patient population is beneficial because it may mean a smaller number of professionals involved in patient care on the unit. A homogeneous population also reduces the number of managed care plans that need to be written. Most units that specialize in certain diseases or surgical procedures will have a smaller physician group with which to interact. A smaller group will allow for a more rapid transition to the model and will be more helpful in formulating the managed care plans because the group will probably be more likely to agree on plans of care.

A greater percentage of high-volume case types will also help when generating managed care plans that will cover a wider number of patients on the unit. In general, if a unit admits more than 50% of its patients to five or fewer DRG categories, the unit may be a good candidate for conversion to case management.

However, it is important to analyze these high-volume case types for their potential in reducing length of stay. High volume does not necessarily mean a reduction in length of stay. For example, some patient problems are on protocols that are already as brief as possible. Chemotherapy is one example. Reductions might not be attainable around the diagnosis, but other elements of hospitalization, such as preadmission blood work or prehydration therapy, may allow for reductions.

The transition to a case management system will require total commitment from those on the unit. One of the most important people in the change process is the nurse manager. The nurse manager has 24-hour responsibility and accountability and has the primary administrative responsibility for the smooth functioning of the unit. Most of the other professionals enter and exit the unit because their responsibilities take them to other areas of the hospital. The nurse manager's sole responsibility is the nursing unit. It is vital that nurse managers have a working knowledge of case management so that they can function both formally and informally as advocates for change. Nurse managers can be instrumental in obtaining the cooperation of physicians with whom they have long-standing relationships.

Most of the activities on a nursing unit revolve around nurse managers who have administrative authority for their units. Their responsibilities may include staffing, budgeting, maintaining supplies, and caring for patients. No changes in these responsibilities should be made without the nurse managers' input and support.

When selecting units for conversion to case management, at least a majority of physicians affiliated with the unit should support the change. This, of course, may not always be possible. Obtaining the support of some physicians can be enough for making a positive transition.

When implementing a case management model, it is helpful but not crucial to begin with a nursing staff that volunteered to be among the first units in the institution to convert. Often, such enthusiasm came from the unit's nurse manager and filtered down to the other nurses on the unit. Again, this may be a factor that is not immediately obtainable.

Most institutions converting to a unit-based model try to do so at minimal cost to the organization. This may mean using an already existing FTE position or a budgeted position that has never been filled. It is not wise to eliminate an employee to make room for a case manager. The open FTE should be acquired through attrition whenever possible because elimination of an employee can cause ill will, resentment, and insecurity among other staff nurses on the unit.

It is often possible to create additional positions once some success has been shown. For these reasons, it is again imperative that the initial units selected indicate a great potential for successful transition.

MEDICAL UNIT

Medical units may possibly be among the neediest in terms of case management patient needs. Medical patients are often elderly and have more complex discharge plans. These patients are often the least likely to be advocates for themselves and are likely to fall through the cracks during an extended and complicated hospital stay. They are among the most costly to hospitals and are often resource intensive.

Medical patients are also among the most difficult to plan for because their hospital course is often unpredictable. Ironically, it is for these reasons that a case manager can be a great asset to a medical unit. The medical patient whose hospital course changes daily needs someone to ensure that everything is happening as planned and that nothing is missed.

There are usually more case managers on a medical unit than on any other type of unit in the hospital. Because of increased complexity and severity of the cases, the organization should aim to have every medical patient under the authority of a case manager. The number of case managers should be based on an average case load of about 15 to 18 patients. If every patient on the medical unit cannot be followed by the case manager, then criteria must be developed for selecting those patients who will benefit the most by being followed. In general, the case load of the case manager on the medical unit must be somewhat smaller than that of either a specialty unit or surgical unit. As stated above, this is because these patients tend to be more resource intensive and the number of interventions per patient will probably be more intense.

Criteria for selecting patients on a general medical floor must be individually determined through a retrospective audit of those patients who seem to represent patterns of increased resource use. However, this is not the only factor that should be evaluated. Other patients who might benefit from a case manager might include those with the following:

- Advanced age (older than 75 years)
- Noncompliance with treatment
- Potential for falls
- Potential for skin breakdown
- Discharge placement problems
- Complicated medical plan

SURGICAL UNIT

Surgical cases can be as complicated as medical cases. Generally, though, the hospital course of a surgical patient is somewhat more predictable and amenable to a predetermined plan. Many surgeons practice with protocols, which manage the patient's postoperative course in the same way that the managed care plan does. Although there are exceptions to every rule, the expected course can be planned around an anticipated length of stay. Surgical patients are often elected admissions, which means that there may be less potential for in-hospital complications.

For these reasons, a surgical case manager may be able to carry a larger patient case load than one on a medical unit. A case load of about 20 patients is probably manageable on most surgical units.

It may not be necessary to have every surgical patient under the direction of a case manager. Criteria for selecting patients should be based on patient need, complexity, or severity of condition. Patients who are admitted for emergency surgery and who require medical clearance before surgery are also some of those who might need the attention of the case manager. Patients who develop postoperative complications, which may result in a prolonged length of stay, should also be considered.

CRITICAL CARE UNIT

The critical care unit may be the last area of the hospital to convert to case management. Because this area has a lower nurse-patient ratio and a more responsive health care team, these patients are already receiving a form of case management.

The case manager and managed care plans may be the only elements missing from these areas. Most intensive care units have a 2:1 or a 1:1 nurse/patient ratio. In these situations it may be possible to use the nurses, in their current positions, to function in a case management role. In this case all registered nurses working in the unit would be case managers. They would be carrying out the functions and responsibilities of the case manager in addition to providing direct patient care.

There are problems with this system, but solutions do exist. The first problem is that continuity of care is still an issue if the unit is on flex time. Also, it may be very difficult for nurses working with critically ill patients to take on the added responsibilities associated with the case manager role. They may not have the time needed to create managed care plans or to be involved in the formation of the team. They may simply be absent from the unit too much to care for patients and function as case managers.

It is possible to create this type of system in critical care areas, but the possible problems must be identified and addressed before implementation. The stress this dual role could impose on the nurses should also be considered.

NURSING HOME

The nursing home is an example of a non-acute care facility that can financially benefit from a case management system. A case management model can ensure a higher quality of patient care with a decreased use of resources. As the population ages and life expectancy increases, the needs of extended-care facilities will rise proportionally. As do most other health care institutions, nursing homes struggle with increased regulations and decreased resources (Smith, 1991).

In the nursing home setting, a case manager can ensure patient outcomes. This can result in a reduced use of registered nurses and an increased use of ancillary personnel.

Nursing homes are required to provide plans of care and goals for their patients. Generally, these plans can be carried out by personnel other than registered nurses. Regulation requires that a registered nurse be present in most instances, but this nurse could be better used as a facilitator, educator, or co-ordinator of services to the patient. This approach can result in enhanced quality of life and slowed deterioration of functional ability.

A team approach with the nurse manager as a case manager can be cost-effective and can ensure improved quality of care. Many institutions have attempted to use the nurse manager in this facilitator role. As in the acute care setting, this dual role has become increasingly difficult in the nursing home setting. By using a case manager, in addition to a nurse manager, greater quality and more efficient clinical outcomes can be achieved.

OUTPATIENT AREA

Case management crosses all boundaries of the health care spectrum. The patient's quality of life may be dependent on the kind of clinical management this person receives in the primary care setting. The approach used in most clinics is a form of case management. Continuity of caregivers is often attempted for a patient's return visits. For many patients without a private family physician, these clinic visits provide their only links to the health care system. Managing patients using the team approach provides for enhanced quality of care.

The future challenge for case management models will be to link the inpatient and outpatient settings in a way that promotes a smooth transition for the patient and ensures continuity of care once the patient returns to the community.

Documentation of the patient's level of compliance after discharge from the hospital can provide valuable data as to the effect hospitalization had on the patient's quality of life. Additionally, a case manager's unique relationship with the patients, as well as follow-up visits and phone calls, can serve as a mechanism for ensuring patient compliance with post-discharge health care follow up.

REFERENCES

Armstrong, D.M., & Stetler, C.B. (1991). Strategic considerations in developing a delivery model. *Nursing Economics, 9*(2), 112-115.

Ethridge, P., & Lamb, G. (1989). Professional nursing case management improves quality, access, and costs. *Nursing Management, 20*(3), 30-35.

Smith, J. (1991). Changing traditional nursing home roles to nursing case management. *Journal of Gerontological Nursing, 17*(5), 32-39.

15

Brainstorming: Development of the Multidisciplinary Action Plan (MAP)

CHAPTER OVERVIEW

The managed care plan is the form of documentation that drives the case management system. Institutions implementing case management models need to determine the form and content of the documentation format they wish to adopt.

This chapter reviews the evolution of managed care plans and the step-by-step process of development. The chapter also discusses the link between the prospective payment system, DRGs, and the managed care plan.

Health care organizations must go beyond what the DRG suggests when designing these plans. The principal procedure or diagnosis should be used with the DRG as the underlying guide for determining the length of the plan.

EVOLUTION OF THE MANAGED CARE PLAN

Just as there are many ways to adapt case management models to fit the needs of a particular organization, there are an infinite number of ways to develop a case management documentation system. Since case managements' inception, most hospitals have been using the *critical path* label on their managed care plans. When introduced in 1985 by the New England Medical Center in Boston, the critical path was the first system that attempted to incorporate expected outcomes within specified time frames. The term *critical path* means that the plan defines the critical or key events expected to happen each day of a patient's hospitalization (Giuliano & Poirier, 1991; Zander, 1991; Zander, 1992).

Since 1985, critical paths have been adapted to meet the needs of organizations implementing case management models. The paths remain an extremely flexible method of planning and documenting. In addition to *critical path* and *critical pathway*, other labels, such as *multidisciplinary plan, multidisciplinary action plan,* and *action plan,* have been attached to these managed care plans. All these

117

terms are the same in theory. Each of the plans attempts to outline the expected outcomes of care for each discipline during each day of hospitalization. Some of these care plans place greater emphasis on the nursing plan, while some emphasize the medical plan of care. Some others, such as the multidisciplinary action plan discussed here, incorporate all disciplines.

Some case management organizations use managed care plans as one-page guides. Essentially these one-page plans are multidisciplinary protocols for the problem or diagnosis. The detail of the plan depends on the goals of the organization in which the plan is being used. In some cases, nursing documentation can be recorded directly onto the form. This format is also easily adapted to a hospital computer system. Computerization of the plan allows the case manager the flexibility of changing the plan as the patient's needs change. For those organizations without a computer system, the managed care plan is still a very easy and flexible tool.

The managed care plan can also be used in place of the traditional nursing care plan. Nursing care plans have been criticized by some as useless exercises in writing. The plans are written to meet the needs of regulatory agencies but are often not used by nurses to guide or plan their day-to-day care. Once written, the plans are often never looked at again. These plans are not even written to provide a plan of care that correlates with the expected length of stay. For this reason these plans are not the preferred form for planning care in case management models.

It is no accident that the critical path or MAP format came into existence. These MAPs are the driving force behind case management models because they help determine the plan of care and arrange that plan around the expected length of stay. Unlike the nursing care plan, MAPs are multidisciplinary and take into account the unique contributions of each discipline. MAPs also link case management with the prospective payment system by using the DRG for determining the appropriate length for the plan. The most current reimbursements are consulted when beginning any plan.

When developing the MAP, keep in mind that the state reimbursable rate may be longer or shorter than the federal rate. Also, it would be impractical to develop standard plans for patients with varying types of insurance coverage. Instead, these variations in reimbursable length of stay can be averaged. Another technique is to determine the length of stay the physician expects and measure it against the reimbursable length of stay. It may turn out that the stay the physician hoped for is shorter than the reimbursable length of stay. In a case like this, the physician's preference would determine the length of stay outlined in the MAP.

However, if the length of stay the physician expects is longer than the reimbursable length of stay, a compromise must be reached. The federal and state rates should be reviewed with the physician in relation to the physician's plan. Areas for reduction should be discussed to reduce the length of stay so that it matches or comes below the reimbursable length of stay. A general guideline is to design the plan so that it is shorter than the reimbursable length of stay. This allows for some margin of error in case the patient requires an additional day of hospitalization.

The case manager can control the length of stay by overseeing the movement of the patient through the system. It is difficult to implement MAPs that will be effective without the position of case manager in place. Instituting plans without a professional to drive the process is not a likely way to achieve the desired results. The staff nurse and the case manager are responsible for ensuring that the expected outcomes, as outlined on the MAP, are carried out. If the expected outcomes cannot be achieved, the case manager analyzes the patient's situation and documents the outcome that cannot be accomplished. This outcome is then documented as a variance, which is anything that does not happen at the time it is supposed to happen.

The DRG must be used as a guide for projecting the length of stay indicated on the MAP. Because the DRG categories are designed for determining hospital reimbursement rates, they are too heterogeneous to assess the effectiveness of the clinical plan at the bedside. For example, if a MAP is written to plan the care of a lumbar laminectomy patient, the discharge diagnosis of lumbar laminectomy might fall under a wide variety of DRGs, such as "medical back procedure" or "spinal procedure." Therefore, if someone wanted to look at the length of stay of all laminectomy patients within a case management system in the hospital, then asking for length of stay records for one DRG would not include the majority of laminectomy patients, who might have been classified under other DRG categories.

Other DRGs are heterogeneous in another way. For example, the DRG for chemotherapy, DRG 410, includes any and all chemotherapy protocols, whether they are for 1 day or for 5 days. The Health Care Finance Administration (HCFA) reimbursement rate for chemotherapy is 2.6 days, regardless of the type of chemotherapy being given. Once again, the DRG system will not be a suitable tool for analyzing whether or not the MAP decreases the length of stay, reduces resource use, or provides the most effective quality care for that problem.

If an organization wants to determine the true effectiveness of managed care plans used among a very specific patient group, the DRG cannot be used. Clinicians must dig deeper, using a microanalysis approach. Patients should be reviewed based on their principal procedure or diagnosis at the time of discharge. This way, the plan's effectiveness can be determined. After all, there is no MAP called "medical back problem," nor can there be one called "chemotherapy" because these would be too general. It follows, therefore, that analysis must be as specific as the level of the diagnosis.

The managed care plan for chemotherapy would be specific to the type of chemotherapy being administered and the specific protocol being followed. In the interest of cost-effectiveness, several chemotherapy protocols can be combined on one MAP. At the time of admission, the patient's specific protocol is identified from a menu of several possible choices on the MAP. All these plans would fall under the same DRG, even though they would be different.

The process for developing the managed care plan must be based on several specific elements. The organization must first decide on the form that the plans will take. Factors that affect the form include degree of complexity, extent to which the plan will include other disciplines, and whether or not the form will include nursing documentation. These factors help determine the plan's design and content. Each factor must be decided before developing the content.

Once the format has been decided and approved, the organization must decide which diagnoses or procedures are to be planned out first. It is obvious that every plan cannot be developed simultaneously. Some general guidelines can be useful in making these decisions. If the model being implemented is a case management, diagnosis-specific approach, then these decisions have probably already been made. Many organizations begin with a few specific diagnoses that are easily planned. Some examples of commonly used diagnoses include "fractured hip," "open heart surgery," and "transurethral prostatectomy" (TURP). These are easily written and followed because these types of procedures are already the subjects of many protocols. It is generally easier to get the cooperation of surgeons who are managing these cases, because they are already managing their patients in a protocol-oriented way. It is also easier to reduce length of stay because the chance of complication or comorbidity is slightly lower in these patient populations than in some others.

If the organization is adopting a unit-based case management model, then deciding which diagnosis to begin with is slightly more complicated although technically the same as for the non unit-based approach. One of the first factors to consider is the number of patients to include in the implementation of one plan. This involves examining the high-volume case types for the organization. Once this is done, an attempt should be made to match these high-volume case types to the units being converted to a case management model. These two factors point to the types of patient problems that should be considered first. After these determinations a match is then made to physicians who work with these patients and who are willing to help develop and adopt managed care plans.

After all these steps have been taken, only then can the actual process of writing begin. There will be several parts to each plan. Generally, the longest of these are the nursing and medical plans. Plans for medical problems are developed from chart review, consultation with experts in the field, and literature review, all to create the "best possible plan" or ideal plan for that patient problem. To make the most of each person's time, individual brainstorming sessions between the case manager and a representative from each discipline are most effective. The case manager can do some preparation to begin the shell of the plan before meeting with anyone. The case manager can determine the approximate length of the plan, based on state and federal reimbursements, and can then begin to plan out the nursing portion of the plan, indicating the expected nursing outcomes for each day of hospitalization.

Once these pieces are complete, the case manager then arranges to meet with members of the other disciplines. The most logical person to begin with is the physician. Plans need to be physician-specific, but this means that several physicians agree as a group to the same plan. Under no circumstances should a completed plan be presented to a physician without first making it clear that the individual preferences and practice patterns of that practitioner will be taken into consideration. Plans should be individualized as much as possible.

Most physicians have a very clear sense of their expectations or of what they would routinely order for the average patient with a particular problem. Of course, not every patient can or will fit into this projected plan exactly. Each plan must be individualized to the patient after admission. The physician should remember that the projected plan is designed for the average patient with a particular problem. This plan could be considered an aggregate of all patients that the physician has treated, discounting unusual or aberrant conditions or circumstances.

On average the plan-development process can be completed in less than an hour. This hour is a small contribution compared with the amount of time it would take for the physician to individually inform all the health care providers of the care plan. Development of a MAP not only saves the physician time but also eliminates the second guessing that sometimes occurs.

One approach for developing a MAP is to simply ask the physician what would routinely be ordered for each day of hospitalization. Systematically running through each day ensures that nothing is neglected. Once all disciplines have completed this process, each should be afforded the opportunity to review the plan one last time. If a group of physicians is involved, each one should have the chance to provide input.

The decision as to which disciplines will be represented in the plan depends on the diagnosis or procedure being planned. For some, physical therapy will be important. For others, respiratory therapy may be necessary. In most institutions social work is a separate component but an integral part of the patient's plan, so this department should be given its own section on every plan. In other institutions some specialties such as skin care nurse, may always be included. The disciplines involved will vary from institution to institution, but in general, nursing, medicine, and social work should be on every plan.

Once each representative has participated in the plan-development process, it would be beneficial to have as many of these people as possible sit down together to review the plan. This form of brainstorming may expose redundant treatments or procedures. This is another significant way of reducing resource utilization, while still providing the best quality of care possible.

MAP TIMELINES

Multidisciplinary action plans can be time-lined in hours, days, weeks, or months depending on the clinical area. Emergency room treatment might be mapped out in terms of hours or parts of an hour. Typical diagnoses, including common medical problems or surgeries, usually fall within a day's time frame. Weeks might be used for those diagnoses that have a longer length of stay, such as those that might be found in a neonatal intensive care unit where the length of stay is three or four months. Month time frames might be relevant in long-term care facilities, such as those for patients with chronic mental disorders, where clinical progress is extremely slow and lengths of stay are measured in years. Nursing home patients provide another example of patient goals that might be evaluated in terms of months.

Once these time frames are determined, variance time frames must be decided.

In other words, when does something become a variance? In what time period should every outcome listed for a particular day be achieved? A variance is anything that does not happen at the time it is supposed to happen. The hospital must decide what kind of leeway will be allowed for achieving these outcomes. Day one will seldom begin at 6 AM on the day of admission because most patients are admitted later in the day. For example, emergency admissions may arrive on the unit in the late afternoon or night shift. It is clear that the beginning and end of any one day in the hospital is a loose concept. Institutions should be generous when deciding on variance time frames. If not, it is possible to set up a situation where almost everything becomes a variance. A plan lasting at least 5 days might not place something into the variance category unless it is not completed within 48 hours.

Documentation of Variances

An area designated for documenting variances should be on the plan. Each variance can be identified and categorized, if desirable. Typical variance categories include the following:
- Operational
- Health care provider
- Patient
- Unmet clinical indicators

An example of operational variances is the breakdown of a piece of equipment, which prevents the completion of a test. Another example is the inability to discharge a patient because no long-term care facilities in the area have an available bed. These are examples of operational variances that go beyond the confines of the hospital. More examples are presented in the box on p. 123.

Healthcare provider variances include any situations in which a health care provider is the cause of the delay in achieving an expected outcome (see the box on p. 123). Discretion must be used when documenting these variances, because some may involve a risk management issue. For example, if the resident is paged several times during the night because a patient has pulled out the nasogastric tube and the resident does not respond for several hours, then the patient misses several doses of medication. Other variances in this category may be associated with the physician's alteration or adjustment of the traditional plan of care.

Patient variances include any patient-related delays (see the box on p. 123). The patient delay may be caused by complications of the patient's medical condition, which require a delay in completion of a test or procedure. For example, the patient may have spiked a fever and may be unable to leave the floor for Magnetic Resonance Imaging (MRI). In other circumstances, the delay may be because the patient refused to have the test or procedure done. Noncompliance frequently causes patient delays. When a patient refuses a test or procedure, the absolute need for the test or procedure should be questioned and evaluated. This sort of stringent review and followup is an example of how a checks-and-balances system in case management can help reduce unnecessary resource use. Tests and

---

OPERATIONAL VARIANCE EXAMPLES

Broken equipment
Lost requisition slips causing delays
Departmental delays due to staffing or other causes
Interdepartmental delays
Larger system delays affecting discharge, such as home care services, equipment, or insurance availability

---

HEALTH CARE PROVIDER VARIANCE EXAMPLES

Deviation from plan due to physician varying the practice pattern
Change related to health care provider's practice patterns, level of expertise, or experience

---

PATIENT VARIANCE EXAMPLES

■ Refusal   ■ Change in status   ■ Unavailability

---

procedures cost the institution money not only in terms of the expense of the supplies and equipment but also in terms of the human resources needed to administer the test and evaluate the results. More timely completion of appropriate tests means a reduction in the length of stay for all patients.

Another patient variance is called *patient variance on admission*. Managed care plans are simple guidelines or expected plans for particular diagnoses or procedures. Regulatory agencies require individualization of any predetermined plans of care during patient admission. This process should be a routine part of putting any patient on a managed care plan. The patient's case should be reviewed in relation to the prewritten plan. Anything different or unusual about the patient's case should yield a change in the plan to make it specific to the patient. One plan is not going to be appropriate for every patient. This process ensures that the plan meets the needs of the patient in question. For example, if the plan calls for a specific medication and the patient is allergic to that medication, the plan should be altered to adjust to that particular patient's clinical condition.

The fourth type of variance is unmet clinical quality indicators (see box on p. 124). Clinical quality indicators are developed in conjunction with the MAP. They are created by the physicians to benchmark clinical outcomes that reflect quality of care rendered. These clinical outcomes can be either intermediate or discharge patient outcomes. The box contains examples of clinical quality indicators that would be developed for asthma team patients.

Variance data are abstracted from the patient's medical record and MAP. The

---

UNMET CLINICAL QUALITY INDICATORS

- Intermediate Outcomes:
   Patient is off IV Solumedrol when Peak Flow > 200
- Discharge Outcomes:
   Peak Flow measurement > 250 L/sec
   Patient is out of bed without shortness of breath
   Patient is able to return demonstration of the use of MDI with spacer

---

analysis of these data is invaluable in determining why an expected patient outcome or clinical quality indicator has not been met. In addition, these data allow for trending of patient outcomes, length of stay, and evaluation of the quality of patient care.

Appendix *1* is an example of a MAP developed and used at the Beth Israel Medical Center in New York City. This MAP is clinically specific not DRG specific. The format illustrated is a preprinted and bound booklet, which outlines the expected outcomes for care for each day of hospitalization for each discipline involved. Medicine, nursing, social work, and discharge planning are automatically included on every plan. Other departments are included as needed. Each department is given a standard place on the form, and content is filled in by members of the discipline during formation of the plan.

The length of the booklet is guided by the reimbursements for the DRGs usually associated with the diagnosis or problem. This information is correlated with what the physician expects the length of stay to be. Generally the physician will adapt to the reimbursement length of stay if this information is supplied in a positive way. If more than one DRG is involved, which is usually the case, then some judgment must be used in determining the shortest possible plan that takes into account the possibly varying reimbursable lengths of stay. In other words, it may be necessary to look at the most commonly used DRGs and follow an average or usual length of stay. Clearly, these expected lengths are "guesstimates" and will not be completely accurate every time. Each plan may be lengthened or shortened depending on patient-related variations but some professional judgment must be used. If a plan is 7 days in length and the patient is ready to go home on the sixth day, an earlier discharge would be completed, and the documentation would be written to reflect the reasons why. A delayed discharge must be documented in the same way with variances that may have resulted in the delay being documented and explained.

During the early phases of DRG use in case management systems, the finer points of the DRG were not always synchronous with the system itself. As the system evolved into more of a financial one, clinical applications of the system needed to remain flexible, and the limitations of such uses needed to be clarified for those clinicians using the system.

Space for nursing documentation has been incorporated into the form of some MAPs. In this space, the registered nurse documents whether or not expected outcomes for the day were achieved and the responses of the patient, when appropriate. Progress notes are included only when a more elaborate or detailed form of documentation is needed, and narrative nurse's notes are eliminated, unless an exception arises. This detailed list of outcomes provides the nurse with an action plan that is specific for that day and keeps the patient on track toward discharge.

For the novice nurse who is less able to project patient needs because of a lack of experience, the MAP provides a plan that is outcome-oriented and guides the new nurse through that particular day of hospitalization. Rather than correcting problems after they have happened, the MAP provides an advanced, detailed plan with tasks that can be carried out in a timely fashion.

The case manager is the driving force behind the success of the managed care plan. It is generally the case manager who checks on variances related to both cause and remedy and who is accountable for the patient's continued success in moving through the system. Using the plan as a guide, the case manager directs all other health care providers toward achieving the expected daily outcome of care.

Another responsibility of the case manager is to provide patient teaching when necessary and to find out why a test or procedure has not been done. The case manager also reviews the care plan with the physician and ensures timely outcomes. Finally, the case manager coordinates with the social worker, discharge planner, family, and patient, to ensure that the best possible discharge plan has been made and that it is ready when the patient goes home. This entire process is communicated to other members of the team through the MAP format and through the case manager's documentation. All in all, the case manager views the whole picture and ensures proper and accurate progress of the patient through the hospital system.

Staff nurses work in collaboration with the case manager and other members of the health care team to ensure that the outcomes of care are achieved within the time frames specified on the MAP. The patient's outcomes are documented by the staff nurse and relate the clinical story of the patient's progress during hospitalization. See the Appendixes for examples of MAPs or critical paths that have been adapted to the needs of various institutions.

REFERENCES

Giuliano, K.K. & Poirier, C.E. (1991). Nursing case management: Critical pathways to desirable outcomes. *Nursing Management, 22*(3), 52-55.

Zander, K. (1991). Care Maps™: The core of cost/quality care. *The New Definition, 6*(3), 1-3.

Zander, K. (1992). Physicians, Care Maps, and collaboration. *The New Definition, 7*(1), 1-4.

METHODS OF EVALUATION

16

The Importance of Research in the Evaluation Process

CHAPTER OVERVIEW

Implementation of a case management model should include establishment of a nursing research methodology. Nursing research data provide the framework for evaluating and justifying the efficacy of the overall model.

This chapter explores methods for designing the research and provides samples for data analysis including patients, staff, and length of stay for selected DRGs. Each organization must determine its own research design based on its goals for the model, but some sort of research base is recommended to provide a framework for evaluation.

DATA TALKS

Someone once said: "In God we trust. When all else fails, use data." Creating change in any organization is never an easy task. Obtaining the support and cooperation of hospital administration is necessary for complete integration of a nursing case management model. With such support the model can be viewed as both a nursing and a multidisciplinary model.

Perhaps the best way to obtain the support of the institution as a whole is through the use of data. This includes collecting, analyzing, and disseminating the results of a statistical data analysis as well as any anecdotal data collected. Some data will already exist and be available in the organization. Other data will need to be collected.

Obtaining administration's support is only part of what is needed as the change to case management proceeds. A sound and valid evaluation process must be implemented to provide ongoing support as the model continues to develop and become part of the institution. It is imperative, therefore, that the elements to be monitored and evaluated are determined before any changes are implemented (Jennings & Rogers, 1986).

Case management provides an opportunity for nursing to conduct research,

129

as well as to quantify the case management model. Research, broadly defined, is an attempt to find the solution to a problem so that it may be predicted or explained (Treece & Treece, 1973). Research has also been described as a formal method for carrying on the scientific method of analysis, which, in turn, involves the use of several problem-solving steps. These include problem identification, hypothesis formation, observation, analysis, and conclusion (Polit & Hungler, 1983).

These basic elements are no less important in the analysis of a case management model and all the changes that come about as a result of the integration of this system (Jennings & Rogers, 1986). Generally, research is divided into two categories. The first is basic research, the goal of which is to obtain knowledge for the sake of knowledge. The second category is applied research which takes this process one step further as it seeks to apply the research to everyday situations (Nachmias & Nachmias, 1981). Case management research is applied research in its truest sense. Everyday questions concerning the efficacy of the model are asked, answered, and applied as the case management research data are collected and analyzed.

The methodology used for case management analysis can take several forms and can encompass several different elements. It need not be limited to one particular process, but can include several steps and processes. Nursing research includes the clinical elements of the nursing profession, such as the steps of the nursing process: assessment, diagnosis, outcome identification, planning, implementation, and evaluation. Nursing research also involves the preparation and evaluation of practitioners and studies the systems in which nurses work and apply the steps of the nursing process (Corner, 1991).

EVALUATION VERSUS EXPERIMENTAL RESEARCH

Research involving case management can be approached as evaluation research. It can also be designed as an experiment or quasi-experiment. In evaluation research, data are collected and analyzed to evaluate or assess the effects of some project or change. This type of research helps to evaluate how well implementation of the program is going.

Experimental research tests the relationships between the variables being manipulated. A control group and an experimental group are used in classic experimental research. The control group symbolizes a normal representation of subjects, and the experimental group consists of those subjects for whom at least one variable has been altered.

In case management research it is difficult to devise a classic experimental design. If patients are compared, the researcher must be sure that the cases are similar enough to justify comparison. Some examples of factors to be controlled when choosing subjects are severity of illness, concurrent problems, gender, and age. In addition, random assignment to each group must be conducted. This process involves the admitting office, which ensures that certain, previously evaluated patients are placed on particular units.

If nurses on nursing units are being studied for job satisfaction, for example, it would be impossible to separate those nurses who had been affected by the model from those who had not. Comparing nurses between nursing units can lead to some of the same methodology questions that arise when comparing some patients with others (Schaefer, 1989). The registered nurses could only be matched if differences were controlled in some way.

Even comparing one nursing unit with another is difficult. There are very few institutions in which nursing-unit patient populations are so similar, and yet so randomized, that nurses' and patients' experiences could be said to be similar from one to the next. It is more likely that comparing one nursing unit with another is like comparing apples with oranges. Nursing units are often designated by specialty, and physicians will usually, whether formally or informally, prefer that patients be sent to a particular nursing unit because the physicians believe that unit is most suited to meeting their patient's nursing needs.

The Quasi-Experimental Approach

Because of the difficulties in matching subjects for control and experimental groups, it becomes practical to use each nursing unit as its own control. Once this takes place, the methodology becomes quasi-experimental. Unit data, including staff satisfaction, length of stay, and so on, are compared before and after implementation. Additional post implementation data are collected and analyzed at predetermined intervals. A longitudinal approach of this kind cannot guarantee that the same staff members will be compared from one time frame to the next (Kenneth & Stiesmeyer, 1991). Whenever possible, the same nurses and staff members should be compared from one time period to the next. For those staff members who come and go during the study, global score comparisons can be made.

Certain intrinsic factors affecting internal validity are impossible to control (Lederman, 1991). One such intrinsic factor that always affects longitudinal studies is maturation. The nurses tested may have either an increase or a decrease in job satisfaction solely because of the passage of time. For some workers, the passage of time provides a certain comfort that increases job satisfaction and sense of accomplishment. For others, longevity can lead to exhaustion, disillusionment, and decreased job satisfaction. In either case, these elements associated with maturation can probably not be controlled.

Another intrinsic factor is that of experimental mortality. While one of the goals of case management is to decrease turnover rates among registered nurses, there will always be a certain amount of turnover among any group of employees, no matter how happy they are with their work. Some may leave because they cannot deal with the changes accompanying the introduction of case management. In either case, it is clear that the researcher will not have the same sample at each stage of data collection. Dropouts from the study can prejudice the results, but, unfortunately, this factor cannot be controlled.

One way to account for the issue of experimental mortality or dropouts is to statistically analyze the entire sample size as a global unit, then match subjects from a previous data collection period with those in the current period and study this group separately.

Subjects serve as their own controls in a pretest-posttest design (Nachmias & Nachmias, 1981). The advantage to this design is that the variable is measured both before and after the intervention. In other words, the variable is compared to itself.

As the first step in either process, preimplementation data and continuous data are obtained as the model goes forward. The provision of a solid nursing research base for evaluation provides credibility to the model for those evaluating it in 6 months, 1 year, 2 years, or longer. (Rogers, 1992).

Typically when changes are made in nursing, very little data collection occurs during the implementation phase (Acton, Irvin & Hopkins, 1991). This lack of data makes validation of results difficult, which, in turn, makes it difficult to maintain the momentum and support needed for change to progress.

To determine what to measure, the organization must first decide what it hopes to achieve by implementing the case management model. After identifying the goal of implementation it will be easier to formulate the questions that should be asked. Based on these questions the researcher can begin to form a hypothesis. The hypothesis indicates what the researcher believes to be the cause and effect of a given situation, and it states the relationship between the variables.

Basic research questions will not be affected by the type of methodology used, regardless of whether an evaluation or experimental methodology is chosen. These research questions are prospective and based on hoped-for outcomes. The outcomes will fall into several categories. Data collection will be longitudinal because it will probably be collected at predetermined intervals over a long period of time. The changes attempted in case management will take years to take hold, so choosing an evaluation time period that is too short may make it appear as if implementation has failed to achieve the desired outcomes. On the other hand, some measure of changing trends will need to be shown within the first year of implementation to prove that things are moving in the desired direction.

The areas affected by the implementation of a case management model are diverse and complicated. They range from patients to staff to finance. Many of the changes are obtuse, intangible, and anecdotal, but others can be validated through stringent data collection and statistical analysis. Those changes to be measured must be determined in advance so that baseline data can be collected. These data will provide the foundation for comparison.

If a case management model is being implemented, the focus of evaluation must be on patients, finance, length of stay, and quality of care.

A nonunit-based case management model is broadly focused, and it may be difficult to prove a relationship between implementation of the model and the level of staff satisfaction. Therefore this might not be a variable worth trying to measure.

In the unit-based case management model, certain changes affect particular nursing staff members in specific ways (Swanson, Albright, Steirn, Schaffner, & Costa, 1992). The response of these individuals can be measured and evaluated in terms of job satisfaction, turnover rates, absenteeism, and vacancy rates.

One of the most difficult but essential elements to measure in a case management model is quality of care. The basic tenet of case management is to move the patient through the hospital system as quickly and efficiently as possible. Because the hospital stay is being accelerated, some controls must be put in place to guarantee that quality care is not being compromised.

Accrediting institutions, such as the JCAHO, are struggling with questions regarding the measurement of quality. These issues will undoubtedly continue into the next century (Williams, 1991).

Perhaps the most tangible measure, and possibly the most important in terms of hospital viability, is the length of stay. Decreases in the length of stay have come to be associated directly with case management. It is difficult to address case management without also addressing the issues of hospital reimbursement and patient length of stay.

The Prospective Payment System has provided the most potent incentive to hospitals to move toward reducing length of stay. These incentives are strictly financial. Shorter hospital stays mean increased profits. It is only a matter of time before every institution in the United States will be looking at measures for reducing length of stay as well as controlling other costs.

Caution should be taken when studying and reporting length of stay statistics. The Prospective Payment System and DRGs were designed to be used only as financial tools for determining reimbursement.

Because of a lack of other ways to tap into this information the DRG has become the basis for studying length of stay and related clinical interventions. A serious analysis of many DRGs will reveal that the DRG is usually too broad and too heterogeneous to be used as a determinant of the effect of a particular clinical intervention.

To report this information with the utmost accuracy, it is more advantageous and appropriate to analyze the situation at a microlevel. For example, there is one DRG for chemotherapy, despite the fact that there are 1-day, 2-day, and 5-day chemotherapy protocols. The reimbursable length of stay is 2.6 days, no matter what the protocol. If a managed care plan is applied to a particular case for a specific chemotherapy protocol in order to determine the effectiveness of the plan, then the researcher would have to identify more than just the DRG. If the plan is a 5-day plan, clearly the reimbursable rate is inadequate. But knowing this information would provide the investigator with an opportunity to determine if the length of stay could have been shortened or if quality care was provided, and so on.

Elements of Data Collection

One form of data collection involves the use of a questionnaire method. By using questionnaires that have been previously determined to be valid and reliable, many of the problems associated with this technique can be reduced or eliminated. The content of the questions determine their ability to control bias, which could influence a respondent's answer in a particular way.

One way to test the staff nurses is to compile packets of various questionnaires

---

DATA COLLECTION MONITORS

1. Improved staff satisfaction
   Outcome indicators:
   a. Registered nurse job satisfaction
   b. Physician job satisfaction
   c. Nursing assistant job satisfaction
   d. Decreased registered-nurse burnout scores
   e. Decreased absenteeism
   f. Decreased turnover rate
   g. Increased recruitment
2. Improved patient satisfaction
   Outcome indicators:
   a. Patient satisfaction
   b. Family satisfaction
3. Improved quality care
   Outcome measures:
   a. Quality assurance data
   b. Patient satisfaction
   c. Readmission rate
   d. Uniform treatment of all cases
   e. Frequency and type of patient education
4. Decreased length of stay
   Outcome measure: reduction in length of stay
5. Improved communication or collaboration among disciplines
   Outcome measures:
   a. Development of collaborative practice groups
   b. Opened lines of communication between all disciplines
   c. Development of managed care plans
6. Decreased costs
   Outcome measures:
   a. Improved resource use (both product and personnel)
   b. Decreased absenteeism, turnover, and vacancy rates
   c. Decreased delays in waiting for tests and procedures
   d. Uniform treatment within physician groups
   e. Alteration of registered nurse and ancillary staff mix

---

including one on demographics, that the researcher can use to describe the sample itself. The questionnaires should take no longer than 15 to 20 minutes to complete (Kenneth & Stiesmeyer, 1991).

The consent form should clearly indicate that participation in the study will in no way affect the respondent's employment in the institution.

When questioning patients, nurses must ensure that patient care is not being disturbed. The researcher must also determine whether or not the patient is able to understand, read, and respond to the questionnaire appropriately. One way to do this is to provide questions on the demographic questionnaire that address the respondent's highest level of education, age, and ability to speak and understand English.

The box on page 134 presents some of the broad categories that an organization converting to a case management model might want to address when collecting data for determining success or failure of implementation.

The list in the above box is certainly not exhaustive. An organization on the brink of implementing case management may choose to study any or all of these questions. Questions may involve a multitude of benchmarks or only a few. There may be areas for study that are not listed in the box but are still very important to the organization in question. Each organization must decide for itself what is most important to measure and how it will be measured. The tools for measuring each of these expected outcomes are determined by the nurse researcher involved in the case management analysis. Valid and reliable tools exist to measure most of the variables, but others will have to be obtained from already-existing hospital information systems, DRG information, and hospital billing records. The areas from which to obtain the data vary from institution to institution. The finance department and the DRG office are two departments that can be of great assistance to the nurse researcher evaluating a case management system. Each unit of analysis will require the use of the nurse researcher's expertise for selecting the most appropriate data with which to answer the research questions.

REFERENCES

Acton, G.J., Irvin, B.L., & Hopkins, B.A. (1991). Theory-testing research: Building the science. *Advances in Nursing Science, 14*(1), 52-61.

Corner, J. (1991). In search of more complete answers to research questions. Quantitative versus qualitative research methods: Is there a way forward? *Journal of Advanced Nursing, 16,* 718-727.

Jennings, B.M., & Rogers, S. (1986). Using research to change nursing practice. *Critical Care Nurse, 9*(5), 76-84.

Kenneth, H.K., & Stiesmeyer, J.K. (1991). Strategies for involving staff in nursing research. *Dimensions of Critical Care Nursing, 10*(2), 103-107.

Lederman, R.P. (1991). Quantitative and qualitative research methods: Advantages of complementary usage. *The American Journal of Maternal/Child Nursing, 16,* 43.

Nachmias, D., & Nachmias, C. (1981). *Research methods in the social sciences.* New York: St. Martin's Press.

Polit, D., & Hungler, B. (1983). *Nursing research.* Philadelphia: J.B. Lippincott Company.

Rogers, B. (1992). Research utilization. *AAOHN, 40*(1), 41.

Schaefer, K.M. (1989). Clinical research: Gaining access to patients. *Dimensions of Critical Care Nursing, 8*(4), 236-242.

Swanson, J.M., Albright, J., Steirn, C., Schaffner, A., & Costa, L. (1992). Program efforts for creating a research environment in a clinical setting. *Western Journal of Nursing Research, 14*(2), 241-245.

Treece, E.W., & Treece, J.W. (1973). *Elements of research in nursing.* St. Louis: The C.V. Mosby Company.

Williams, A.D. (1991). Development and application of clinical indicators for nursing. *Journal of Nursing Care Quality, 6*(1), 1-5.

17

Documentation of Quality Care

CHAPTER OVERVIEW

For health care organizations to improve delivery of services, they must first determine their definition of quality. Recently, quality issues have moved from an organizational perspective to a consumer-oriented one, in which the needs and concerns of the customer count.

Among the elements measured in defining quality is patient satisfaction. Patients can be questioned directly through focus groups or indirectly through written questionnaires.

Each organization must determine its measures in relation to the incorporated case management documentation system. Patient, health care provider, and operational variances can be used to continuously improve quality. The case manager serves an important role in this process.

WHAT IS QUALITY?

The meaning of quality takes on a new twist when introduced as a concept relevant to health care. Quality may be seen in terms of its effect on the health care delivery system or on specific dimensions of the system (Institute of Medicine, 1976).

On the larger scale of the entire health care system, quality may include the following: availability and accessibility of health care services, credentialing requirements and standards of the providers, comprehensive assessment and documentation, collaborative and informed relationships with the patient and family, minimal injuries or complications to hospitalized patients, evaluation of new technology and resources, and effective management of health care resources (McCarthy, 1987).

The advent of the Prospective Payment System forced health care institutions to focus on health care as a business. Leaving good-quality care to chance did not work and ultimately did not make good business sense. As organizations, regulatory agencies, and patient needs became more complicated, it became ob-

136

vious that health care was no less a business than any other and that the product of the business was patient care. Increasingly, the value of that care became dependent on the matching of cost and quality. Before determining the value of the product, organizations first needed to know what the expected quality would be.

Manufacturers, small-business owners, and large corporations have known for years that in order to provide quality, the organization or business must first determine its definition of quality (Davis, 1990). Discovering what attributes the organization wants to attain is one way to arrive at such a definition.

Health care organizations have already begun to realize that a change in the definition and measurement of quality is needed (Jones, 1991). The products of health care are often intangible items that are difficult to identify and measure. Quality assurance measures in the past have attempted to identify errors and then place blame on the individual who made the error. However, one could argue that counting the number of bedsores or medication errors does not help define quality health care.

Consumer Focus

As in business, it became obvious that one useful technique for defining quality health care was to ask the recipients of that care. This technique of asking consumers what they want often highlights issues to which the health care practitioner is blind. In the past, our definition of quality was to count the number of patient falls. If the organization came in below the desired threshold, it was providing quality care. However, the patient's definition of quality was care given by a competent, pleasant employee who was familiar with the patient and the patient's needs.

Of course, the issue of falls is an important one in terms of assuring quality, and patients will surely consider this equally important if they have ever fallen. The point is, that once the customer's needs have been queried and identified, an entirely new area can be addressed. Invariably, the necessary dimensions of quality that the consumer identifies focus on the business end of health care. This area has been ignored in the past. Organizations believed they knew what patients needed and supplied it to them within the constraints and needs of the organization. The patient had to conform to the organization. There are occasions when this approach is truly necessary. But remaining forever in this mind set eliminates the possibility of ever going beyond providing basic services, and it certainly does not allow for an atmosphere of continual improvement.

By determining what constitutes quality, it can be measured. Once measured, it can be managed. Managing care allows for a process of continual improvement toward excellence, and excellence is the definition of quality.

PATIENT SATISFACTION

With a renewed focus on patient needs, the issue of how to measure patient satisfaction has never been more important. Patient satisfaction is quickly becoming the benchmark for measuring quality health care. Customer needs are not only identified but also form the basis from which quality improvements are made. Within the mission statement of most health care oganizations is a clause that cites patient satisfaction as a goal. Although the health care industry has always identified itself as a serivce industry, clearly this was a self-serving need. In most instances the attitude of health care providers was that the patient was lucky to be getting what they were getting.

How often have nurses used the following phrases in defense of a system that was obviously failing the patients and customers?

"You had to wait five days for a CAT scan? Well, Mrs. Jones had to wait six days. Aren't you lucky?"

"You haven't seen your surgeon since the operation? That is something you are going to have to accept if you want to have the very best surgeon in this field."

The patients were certainly not lucky to be sick, to be in the hospital, or to be having surgery. When even minimal expectations are not being met, then something is terribly wrong with the system.

Customer service will be what defines quality in the next century. Health care organizations that provide service to all customers, from physicians to patients to the community, will be the most successful. The focus must shift away from a purely organizational approach to one that blends consumer and organizational needs (Strasen, 1991).

Depending on the philosophy, resources, and goals of the organization, the approach for measuring patient satisfaction can be made in a number of ways.

Generally, a questionnaire is used to gauge the level of patient satisfaction. Such a survey can be administered while the patient is in the hospital or after discharge (Steiber & Krowinski, 1990). Generally, an attempt is made to administer the questionnaire 24 to 48 hours before discharge. However, some patients may be intimidated by a questionnaire that is filled out while they are still in the hospital, fearing that if a bad report is given, one of the health care providers may retaliate with less than optimal care.

On the other hand, patients' memories of their hospital stays will be most vivid if recorded while still in the hospital. Positive and negative impressions will be fresh in their minds, and these impressions can provide valuable information.

However, patients who are queried after discharge, in the safety and comfort of their homes, may be more likely to provide honest information because they have no fear of retribution. Unfortunately, positive and negative experiences can be quickly forgotten once the patient is home, which means valuable information can be lost if patients are questioned in this manner.

The pros and cons of each method must be evaluated by each organization. There is no perfect way, and it is possible that some form of patient-satisfaction questioning is already in place. These data can be used both as preimplementation data and for ongoing studies.

If the questionnaires are administered to patients while they are in the hospital, someone who is not directly involved in the care of the patient should administer the survey to the patient. This method will help to diminish potential for bias.

Because people who are ill or who have recently been ill are being questioned, care should be taken to select a questionnaire that has short, understandable questions. The focus of each question should be clear to the patient. Patients who are questioned while still in the hospital are more likely to be experiencing increased anxiety or other physical conditions that may affect their abilities to participate.

It is best to select instruments that have been previously identified as valid and reliable. Most instruments use closed-ended questions in which a series of possible choices are given. This format is easiest to score and analyze statistically. Open-ended questions provide the investigator with less control of response content and are more difficult to analyze. Even so, the open-ended format may provide the most meaningful information. It may be beneficial to design an instrument that combines both close-ended as well as open-ended questions. This allows for some control over responses and the opportunity to elicit useful anecdotal information.

The focus of the survey may also depend on the philosophy and goals of implementing the case management system. Many patient satisfaction surveys focus on hygiene needs, such as food, room comfort, noise, and so on. Although these factors are important, they may not be capturing the elements that a case management system is attempting to change. Therefore, it may be necessary to find a questionnaire that focuses more on the professional care provided. In some cases, the institution may have to develop its own instrument that clearly questions the patients in regard to this unique switch to case management.

Developing an instrument can be difficult. The decision to develop a unique questionnaire should not be taken lightly. If the organization is looking for immediately valid and reliable results, the use of a pilot instrument is not the best route to take. The use of more than one instrument is one way to address this dual need so that the needs of both the organization and the researcher can be met. Previously established questionnaires allow for a rapid compilation of information with which to measure implementation. However, in the long run, a new questionnaire, aimed at determining specific effects of the case management system on the patient, will contribute a great deal to the validation of the model's efficacy. In addition the questionnaire can be used by other organizations that implement case management systems.

Another technique is the qualitative method. Qualitative assessment is used to compile data that can be used later in a self-report or paper-and-pencil questionnaire. Patient-focused groups and interviews provide data for development of written questions. Qualitative approaches allow the researcher to see the situation through the experience of the patient. The perceptions of the patient are used to compile information that is later categorized. These categories are then transformed into specific questions.

The qualitative method is very time-consuming. Personal interviews or focus groups last from 1 to 2 hours, but the researcher has to devote even more time to use this form of data collection. However, the information gained can be invaluable.

Determining which patients to question is really a matter of good research technique. The sample should be as heterogeneous as possible to allow for the greatest deal of generalizability. Random sampling will provide this.

Every health care organization compiles statistics that are fed back to regulatory agencies. This information is generally used to determine accreditation and licensing, and to analyze mistakes, untoward effects, and outcomes. Information categorizing the number and type of falls, infections, and medication administration errors has been tracked for years. Analysis of these data helps identify patterns or frequent offenders. Such a system has been referred to as the "bad apple" approach. If a health care practitioner makes a mistake, then that person is counseled. If the practitioner makes the same kind of mistake repeatedly, more serious intervention on the part of the employer might take place. This system does not take into account possible system issues that may contribute to the problem. Instead, one person is seen as the cause of the problem as well as the means for fixing it.

This approach not only looks for the bad apple but also lies in wait for the accident or error. The approach does not provide a mechanism for addressing the larger elements of the problem, and it does nothing to control the recurrence of this problem.

Nevertheless, most institutions evaluating case management systems have turned to the bad-apple approach in an attempt to prove quality patient care. A reduction in patient falls or patient infections might be reported as a result of the introduction of a case management model. In reality, the factors leading to a fall or an infection go beyond a managed care plan or a case manager.

If the goal of data analysis is to improve the quality of care, then a method other than the bad-apple approach must be selected. Patient care is simply too multidimensional to be analyzed effectively by this method. Identifying more appropriate data to measure will come as a direct result of establishing a definition of quality. Case management data is positive outcome data because it focuses on the expected outcomes of the interventions in which we participate as health care providers. The managed care plan provides all the expected outcomes of care during hospitalization, from patient teaching expectations to expected resource use to expected length of stay.

These expected outcomes provide the foundation for determining quality care. By delineating these outcomes, each discipline is identifying the quality issues around a particular diagnosis or procedure.

Additional indices of patient's perceptions of quality can be identified. These indicators should be incorporated into any measure of quality. Until the organization has converted to a case management system or until the new managed care plans are in place, it may be necessary to continue to report the quality assurance data to obtain baseline indices of quality. Ultimately, this format can be abandoned or combined with other quality indicators.

CRITERIA FOR MEASURING OUTCOMES

Some of the outcomes identified on the managed care plan can be tracked during hospitalization. These outcomes are the day-to-day clinical, psychosocial, and teaching interventions identified on the plan. The case manager addresses these on a daily basis and ensures that the patient is moving along the continuum of health care in a timely fashion. If any outcome is not achieved, the case manager is responsible for determining why and correcting the problem or changing the plan.

The unit of analysis within the managed care plan will vary depending upon the increments in which the hospital stay is measured. For example, while most managed care plans are developed on the basis of the 24-hour day, others may have longer or shorter units of analysis. In the neonatal intensive care unit, where the expected length of stay can run from 1 to 3 months, daily measures are not appropriate. In this case, the managed care plans are "time-lined" in 1-week intervals, during which the expected outcomes should be achieved.

In some cases, such as an emergency room setting, the time frames may be very short. In these cases, the managed care plan time frames are set at 15-minute or 30-minute intervals. During these shorter time periods, very specific outcomes are expected. Whatever the time frame, it should realistically correlate to the clinical situation being planned. Once a unit of analysis or time period is chosen, analysis can begin.

In case management anything that does not happen when it is supposed to happen is called a variance. Variances alert practitioners to changes in the patient's condition, or they highlight problems in the health care delivery system itself. Any variances that occur are identified daily as well as retrospectively. Every expected outcome on the plan is a potential variance, and, unless the outcome is achieved within a predetermined time period, it falls into the variance category. As outlined in Chapter 15, there are four causes for variances: the patient, the health care provider, operations or unmet clinical indicators.

There are two types of patient variances. The first is a patient variance or condition identified on admission. These conditions may or may not require an alteration in the usual plan for that diagnosis or procedure. For example, a patient allergy identified at the time of admission might mean that a drug usually considered standard for that diagnosis or procedure cannot be administered. As a result, the plan of care must be discussed with the physician who decides either to refrain from using the drug or to replace it with a suitable alternative.

In some cases the variance is noted, but no change is made to the plan at that time. An example of this is a patient who has diabetes. The person admitting this patient reviews the plan and notes that no changes are needed. The patient's condition still needs to be noted in the Patient Variance on Admission section of the managed care plan. This alerts all health care providers that the patient has diabetes. It also indicates that the plan was individualized at the time of admission.

The other type of patient variance is one that the patient causes. In other words, this type involves situations in which an expected outcome cannot be achieved because of the patient's condition or noncompliance.

For example, a tuberculosis managed care plan might call for collection of sputum specimens on the first, second, and third days of hospitalization. If the patient is unable to produce sputum on the second day, that outcome cannot be achieved within the anticipated time frame. In such a case, specimen collection is moved to the third and fourth days.

An example of a patient variance caused by noncompliance might occur on the second postoperative day, when the plan calls for the patient to dangle his legs over the edge of the bed. Because of pain, the patient refuses. Despite pain medication, the patient continues to refuse. This refusal results in an inability to achieve the desired outcome, and the patient's plan has to be adjusted accordingly.

By reviewing the patient's progress throughout the day and anticipating the course of recovery for the entire hospital stay, the case manager can adjust the plan so that the variance does not change the length of stay. If the patient refuses to ambulate, then the "dangling" and "out-of-bed-to-the-bathroom" goals can be combined into expected outcomes for the following day, when the patient is feeling better. Another possibility might be to try the dangling step again on the next shift, when the pain medication is more effective.

Regardless of the reason for the variance, the case manager and the staff nurse should be aware of the recovery protocol and should attempt to get the patient back on track as soon as possible. This method helps avoid unnecessary delays and makes the patient's progress and expected plan well-known and easily tracked. This in turn means that potential problems will be less likely to continue for several days without being noticed.

A health care provider variance is caused by an omission or error made by a health care practitioner. Institutions have unique regulations regarding documentation, and employees must acquaint themselves with these policies. However, mistakes are bound to occur.

An example of a health care provider variance might involve a transcription error. If a physician order for a medication is not transcribed by the nurse, but the error is detected on the next shift, then the patient might have missed a dose of the medication. Other health care provider variances involve changes in practice patterns that cause the patient's plan to deviate from the predetermined managed care plan.

Operational variances are probably the most commonly occurring variances. Operational variances include those that happen within the confines of the hospital as well as some that can occur as a result of some condition outside the hospital.

A large-system variance, one that occurs because of something outside the hospital, might involve discharge placement. These types of variance would fall within the operational category. Sometimes a patient is assessed as appropriate for nursing home placement, so all the paper work is completed, and the patient is clinically ready for discharge, but no nursing-home beds are available. As a result, the patient remains in the hospital until a bed becomes available, and the extended stay is classified as a large-system variance.

The most typical kinds of large-system variances usually involve postdischarge problems in which a proper discharge location is not available. This type of variance is difficult to control. The best prevention is for the case manager to attempt to identify those patients who will need placement as early in the hospital stay as possible and begin to prepare the necessary paperwork so that delays can be avoided.

Other operational variances can occur because of the institution's infrastructure. Most health care institutions are large, complex places. Systems have developed over time, often without planning. Once these systems are in place, most workers are too busy to correct the operational problems. Instead, informal mechanisms are developed to work around the flaw in the system.

These kinds of operational problems can delay the patient's progress toward discharge. An inadequate patient-scheduling system may mean that the nursing unit is unaware of a scheduled procedure, and the patient is not correctly prepped. This results in an inability to complete the procedure and may mean an increase in the length of stay.

Other operational variances occur when equipment breaks. One such operational variance is an inability to complete a CT scan because the machine is not functioning. Any equipment malfunction results in a delay, which, in turn, takes the patient off the managed care plan schedule. Clinical quality indicators are those expected clinical indicators identified by the physician that may include intermediate and discharge outcomes. These indicators are used to assess clinical progress and quality of care. See Chapter 15 for more information on variances.

Any of these variances require the input of the case manager whose responsibility is to identify the variance and intervene to correct it. The goal is to minimize the effect the variance will have on the patient's length of stay.

The other responsibility of the case manager is to document the variance. Retrospective analysis of operational variances results in the identification of frequently occurring, but rectifiable, problems. It is important that variances also be documented for the purposes of utilization review and reimbursement.

REFERENCES

Davis, W.W. (1990). Quality care and cost control? *The Case Manager, 1*(3), 24-29.

Institute of Medicine. (1976). Assessing quality in health care: An Evaluation. (DHEW Publication No. 282-75-0437 PM). Washington, D.C.: National Academy of Sciences.

Jones, K.R. (1991). Maintaining quality in a changing environment. *Nursing Economics, 9*(3), 159-164.

McCarthy, C. (1987). Quarterly health care inches closer to precise definition. *Hospital Peer Review,* (Feb.), 19-20.

Steiber, S.R. & Krowinski, W.J. (1990). *Measuring and managing patient satisfaction.* Chicago: American Hospital Publishing.

Strasen, L. (1991). Redesigning hospitals around patients and technology. *Nursing Economics, 9*(4), 233-238.

18

The Link Between Continuous Quality Improvement and Case Management

CHAPTER OVERVIEW

During the past several years, the continuous quality improvement (CQI) process has gradually been adapted to the health care setting to improve quality without increasing costs. In traditional quality assurance models, quality is measured by the number of accidents or errors occurring. No provision is made for improving the conditions under which the errors occurred.

However, continuous quality improvement focuses on the processes used to achieve a goal. These processes may be clinical, financial, or operational issues. Each step in the process is analyzed; then, a plan for improvement is tested and refined.

The three leaders in the CQI process are Deming, Juran, and Crosby. Each has made unique contributions toward improving the quality of work performed in the industrial setting. Now their concepts are being applied in the health care arena.

Case management and CQI are linked in philosophy and process. The steps of the CQI process can be applied to managed care plans from both clinical and financial perspectives.

INTRODUCTION TO CONTINUOUS QUALITY IMPROVEMENT (CQI)

The CQI process was officially introduced in 1991 as a more effective approach to improving the quality of health care. In that year the JCAHO announced that it would be introducing new standards requiring all chief executive officers of hospitals to be educated on CQI methods (Hospitals, 1991). This mandate went into effect for accreditation surveys as of January 1, 1992.

This seemingly abrupt switch from traditional quality assurance methods to an approach that had had tremendous success in the business arena was timely. Quality had become the promotional tool for many health care organizations as they adopted a more consumer-oriented approach (Naisbitt, 1982).

At the same time, the prospective payment system had changed the speed and scope of health care delivery. Techniques that had been successful in the past were no longer financially feasible. Change, once considered something to be avoided, was hailed as the way to financial viability for the industry (Kanter, 1983). The changes included new and more effective management styles, which could provide quality under a cost-containment umbrella.

Another force driving the need for change was an emerging consumerism (Naisbitt, 1982). The average person had become an educated health care consumer and was more expectant of quality care. Consumers wanted to be involved in their care, which included participation in decisions involving treatment, cost, and self-care (O'Connor, 1984).

Continuous quality improvement falls in the realm of total quality management, a concept originated by W. Edward Deming (Hospital Peer Review, 1988). Quality improvement involves an analysis, understanding, and improvement of the processes of care. In the case of the health care industry, these processes include the hospital system, the personnel, the clinical management, and financial structure that surround each patient case.

In this format, quality is defined as the meeting or exceeding of customer requirements (Marszalek-Gaucher & Coffey, 1990). In other words, the customer defines quality. Suppliers and customers are involved in each of the above mentioned processes. The supplier is the one who passes on the patient, information, or equipment, and the customer is the one who receives the patient, information, or equipment.

One of the first steps in CQI is the identification and study of the individual steps that make up each of the processes of health care. This CQI extends beyond individual departments because the exchanges between departments are usually the areas that yield difficulties. Each process can be broken down into its working parts in a variety of ways. One way is with the use of a flow chart. The flow chart pictorially describes each step and is useful in helping to identify where bottlenecks or overuse of resources are occurring. Figure 18-1 is a simplified example of how a CT scan scheduling process is broken down into its major steps.

Root causes of problems are identified through the flow chart. Once the root causes have been determined, more data can be gathered, and the team can begin selecting solutions. It is necessary to pick the root cause that may result in the greatest initial improvement of the process. Additional causes can then be addresssed, after one solution has been tried. At this point, more data should be collected to evaluate whether the solution was given enough time to take hold and whether it was effective.

TRADITIONAL QUALITY ASSURANCE

The health care industry has been crippled by waste and misuse of resources (Marszalek-Gaucher & Coffey, 1990). Within this wasteful environment, quality care has always been difficult to measure (Goldfield & Nash, 1989). Compounding this difficulty is the unabated growth of industry inspection, which has resulted

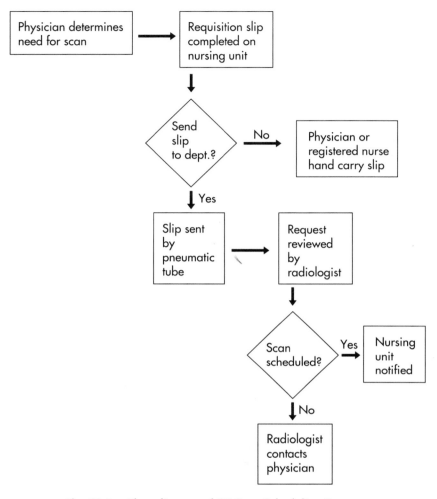

Fig. 18-1 Flow diagram of CT Scan Scheduling Process.

in an adversarial relationship between health care organizations and inspection agencies. Sanctions mandating quality as defined by agencies, such as the Peer Review Organizations (PRO), the JCAHO, the state licensing agencies, and others, have resulted in measures designed to ensure minimum expectations rather than continuous improvement (Laffel & Blumenthal, 1989).

Relatively arbitrary thresholds have been established within organizations. These thresholds define minimum expectations and identify bad apples, but do not provide any mechanism for finding causes or suggestions for improvements. These techniques for assuring quality do not address health care's increasing need for improvement in all processes of the industry (Donabedian, 1980). It is clear that while quality has to be maintained, systems have to be designed for improving business at all levels.

The traditional quality assurance process provides a system for identifying opportunities to improve care or problems. These opportunities are based on the collection of information on incidents or errors, which have surpassed a predetermined threshold (see the box on page 148). Factors affecting the occurrence of the incidents, the systems affecting the errors, or processes for improvement are not identified.

In addition, errors or incidents are identified through individual finger-pointing based on the mistake of one person. Therefore, each quality issue appears to be the fault of one particular person, acting independently. This focus removes all accountability from the organization or the systems within which the individual practitioner is working.

THE NEW HEALTH CARE AGENDA

Quality has become paramount on the health care agenda. Industrial models of quality improvement have been adopted and used successfully in the health care arena. Industry's goals, the reduction of costs and the improvement in the quality of the product, match those of health care. More than a decade ago, industrial leaders realized that to compete and survive in a world economy, quality improvement techniques were needed, which would yield significant operational improvements (Drucker, 1991; Hickman & Silva, 1984; Naisbitt & Aburdene, 1985; Tichy & Devanna, 1986).

The three individuals most closely associated with these processes are Philip B. Crosby, W. Edwards Deming, and Joseph M. Juran.

Crosby is probably the best known of the three quality experts. His approach is based upon his *Fourteen Steps* for the Quality Improvement Process (QIP) (Crosby, 1979).

1. Management commitment
2. Quality improvement team
3. Measurement
4. Cost of quality
5. Quality awareness
6. Corrective action
7. Zero defects planning
8. Employee education
9. Zero defects
10. Goal setting
11. Error cause removal
12. Recognition
13. Quality councils
14. Do it all over again

Crosby (1979) explains that his efforts are different from those of Juran or Deming in that these *Fourteen Steps* provide a complete process. This process, says Crosby, provides a methodology for improving quality, not just a series of quality improvement techniques.

W. Edward Deming is the leading figure in quality improvement. It was Dem-

---

QUALITY ASSURANCE MONITORING AND EVALUATION
THE TEN STEP PROCESS

1. Assign responsibility for monitoring and evaluating activities.
2. Delineate the scope of care provided by the organization.
3. Identify the most important aspects of care provided by the organization.
4. Identify indicators (and appropriate clinical criteria) for monitoring the important aspects of care.
5. Establish thresholds (levels, patterns, trends) for the indicators that trigger evaluation of the care.
6. Monitor the important aspects of care by collecting and organizing the data for each indicator.
7. Evaluate care when thresholds are reached in order to identify either opportunities to improve care or problems.
8. Take actions to improve care or to correct identified problems.
9. Assess the effectiveness of the actions and document the improvement in care.
10. Communicate the results of the monitoring and evaluation process to relevant individuals, departments, or services, and to the organization-wide quality assurance program.

Copyright 1990 by the Joint Commission on Accreditation of Healthcare Organizations, Oakbrook Terrace, IL. Reprinted with permission.

ing who, working with Japanese manufacturers in the 1950s, was responsible for the tremendous improvements made in Japanese manufacturing. To make improvements, Deming relies on technical expertise as well as statistical analysis. His work helped place the Japanese in a completely different class of manufacturing.

Deming's (1986) approach places emphasis on "Fourteen Points," which have been used in the transformation of American industry:

1. Create constancy of purpose for improvement of product service.
2. Adopt a new philosophy.
3. Cease dependence on inspection to achieve quality.
4. End the practice of awarding business on the basis of price tag alone. Instead, minimize total cost by working with a single supplier.
5. Improve constantly every process for planning, production, and service.
6. Institute training on the job.
7. Adopt and institute leadership.
8. Drive out fear.
9. Break down barriers between staff areas.
10. Eliminate slogans, expectations, and targets for the work force.
11. Eliminate numerical quotas for the work force and numerical goals for management.
12. Remove barriers that rob people of pride of workmanship. Eliminate the annual rating or merit system.
13. Institute a vigorous program of education and self-improvement for everyone.
14. Put everybody in the company to work to accomplish the transformation.

Deming (1986) may be best known for his work in involving the employee in the quality improvement system. Concepts such as the "quality circle" or the "QC circle" grew out of the development of these processes, which involved groups of employees in problem identification and solving. Perhaps most relevant in adapting Deming's work to the health care industry is its focus on implementing intervention strategies to improve quality and reduce cost. Other aspects applicable to health care are the continuous improvement in quality, and the use of employee teams trained in problem-solving techniques (Deming, 1986).

Juran was with Deming in the 1950s in Japan and had previously worked with Deming in the 1920s at the Hawthorne Western Electrical Plant in Chicago. Juran, like Deming, is considered a pioneer and an expert in quality improvement technology. Best known for his *Quality Trilogy*, (Juran, 1987, 1988) Juran broadened the quality approach to a wider operational/managerial perspective.

Quality Planning—The process of developing the products and processes required to meet customer needs.

Quality Control—The regulating process through which actual performance is measured and compared to standards and the difference is acted upon.

Quality Improvement—The organized creation of beneficial change.

The structure, process, and outcome approaches of these quality issues can be operationalized and evaluated for continuous improvement. With the patient as focus, quality is identified as those factors most important to patient and family. If asked, the patient might identify many of the factors outlined in Figure 18-2 as important to care.

THE LINK TO CASE MANAGEMENT

Data for analysis in traditional quality assurance methods have focused on "un-quality" or "disquality," such as infections, falls, medication errors, returns to the operating room, and deaths.

Some of these elements focus on the institution, such as global indicators of quality within the hospital. Examples of global indicators include morbidity and mortality rates and generic risk-management indicators. The focus of these elements has been on those identified as outliers.

Another traditional data base has been financial data and analysis, which tracks the cost of specific procedures, or DRGs. The finance department uses this information to determine case mix index, which in turn helps determine the reimbursement rate.

Data related to individual practitioners have been more loosely followed. Utilization review evaluators and other quality management departments have focused on specific practice patterns.

Within case management, each of these elements can be followed more comprehensively. The data, once collected, are linked to continuous quality improvement methods. The first step in a CQI process such as this is to identify problems that appear to be more than isolated events, and to identify all of the issues that may be affecting the outcome. These issues might be linked to a DRG cost analysis

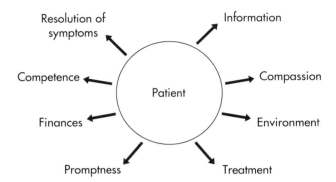

Fig. 18-2 Patient Care Concerns, Courtesy A. Ron and M. Holtz. Beth Israel Medical Center, 1992.

as well as to individual practice patterns. In a case management framework, all practitioners are monitored for quality, use of resources, and length of stay.

The managed care plan is the foundation for this kind of data collection and analysis. The managed care plan provides a guideline for administering care to a particular patient type. These plans take into consideration not only length of stay but also resource use. During the development of the managed care plan, the most optimal treatment plan, one that streamlines care without compromising quality, is identified.

If planned correctly, these collaborative guidelines are agreed upon by the group of practitioners for whom the guidelines are relevant. These plans, in essence, describe the one best treatment plan for a particular patient problem. By following these guidelines, quality issues are easily tracked. The managed care plan provides the collection and evaluation of variances or complications or both. These data may or may not reveal the need to alter the plan to improve quality (Deming, 1986).

For example, a plan for the treatment of pneumonia may indicate that more than 50% of the patients managed by this plan develop some complication on the third or fourth day. This pattern is seen when retrospectively analyzing the variances documented on the managed care plan. A review of this information may indicate the need for a change in the protocol. This may mean providing some element of the plan either earlier or later in the hospital stay.

The cost of the hospital stay can also be followed through the use of the managed care plans. Performance within a particular DRG can be tracked financially, through a quality perspective, or both. Comparing case-managed patients to similar patients who are not case managed is one way to do this tracking. Another method is to compare physicians' practice patterns and any deviations from the care plan. This information then can be evaluated for both quality and cost.

Monitoring length of stay and/or cost before and after implementation of the case management system allows particular nursing units to be their own controls.

If nursing documentation is a part of the managed care plan, the documentation is reviewed for completeness. The registered nurse documents against each expected outcome as it appears on the plan. Thus the documentation more accurately reflects the plan of care and the expected outcomes.

In any case, the processes surrounding the quality issue become the main focus when using a CQI approach. Theoretically, this process makes continuous analysis and improvement possible because it pinpoints every imperfection in the process and opens the door for change (Berwick, 1989).

THE COST OF QUALITY

Poor quality is costly (Marszalek-Gaucher & Coffey, 1990), and can be assessed by the following:
- Cost associated with giving wrong medications or treatments
- Increased costs related to misuse of personnel/product resources
- Cost of delays
- Loss of sales because of dissatisfied patients or physicians

Crosby stresses a "cost of quality" determination as part of the quality improvement process (Quest for Quality, 1989). His outline parallels actions used when developing a managed care plan. However, the development of the managed care plan takes Crosby's process one step further, because it addresses issues and incorporates solutions into the plan of care. Crosby describes the issues and solutions as the following:
- Audit medical records to determine medically unnecessary tests, treatments, or procedures and other factors contributing to increased cost or length of stay.
- Meet with a quality assurance/utilization review representative and review incident reports to determine opportunities for improvement.
- Interview key members of the organization to identify barriers to the smooth operation and coordination of care.
- Interview the medical staff to identify areas for improvement.
- Review and analyze patient records to identify costs that can be eliminated.
- Evaluate current reporting procedures, information related to operations, and data related to patient satisfaction.

The cost-of-quality analysis provides for the identification of a number of potential opportunities for quality improvement. From a case management perspective, the information may provide the foundation for managed care plans by taking into account the best, most cost-effective method available.

THE CQI PROCESS

The CQI process consists of a number of specific steps. Although it is not necessary to follow the steps in a precise sequence, all steps should be evaluated and addressed (Marszalek-Gaucher & Coffey, 1990). The achievement of quality care and cost savings is the foundation of both case management and CQI. The process is a cycle, which continuously repeats itself.

As with the case management implementation process, the first major step in the CQI process is that of planning and preparing to improve; the second step is to implement; the third step is to innovate.

Preparing to improve involves seven essential steps (Marszalek-Gaucher & Coffey, 1990). Once again, it is not necessary to follow them in precise order, but each should be addressed in some manner:

1. **Find a process.** The first step is to find a process that needs quality improvement, cost control, or both. These processes may be within a clinical, operations, or financial setting from admitting, to medication distribution, or billing.
2. **Assemble a team that knows the process.** It has been said that those who know the process best are those working the front line or those who work within the process on a day-to-day basis. Therefore a large percentage of the team should be those directly involved in health care delivery. Management should also be included, because this division can remove obstacles and facilitate change and improvement. In any case, the members of the team should know the process they are evaluating.
3. **Identify the customers and the process outputs, and measure the customer expectations of these outputs.** Quality has been defined as meeting or exceeding customer expectations (Hospital Peer Review, 1988). Because of the complexity of health care, each process may be made up of several smaller processes. The first thing the team should do is identify its customers, the outputs of each process and customer expectations regarding these outputs. In some cases, such as clinical settings, the expectations may not be those of individuals but of the profession as a whole. These expectations may be based on professionwide standards for the practice of nursing and medicine.
4. **Document the process.** Each process consists of a series of steps or inputs, each of which is working toward a particular output. Each step can usually be broken down into substeps, which are hierarchical. A fundamental knowledge of the process is necessary to identify each of the steps accurately, and this is why the input of the front-line worker is so important. A process cannot be managed or improved without this fundamental knowledge.
5. **Generate output and process specifications.** Specifications are measurable, explicit attributes expected of the process and the output. Output specifications may involve the expectations of the customers, which are considered expectations external to the process. However, process specifications are the key internal process factors.

    Each of the specifications must be measurable. When these specifications are achieved, quality is achieved. Quality is maintained by conforming to these specifications, which is precisely what the managed care plan facilitates. The expected outcomes, if met, ensure quality care has been delivered for that particular problem. As these processes and outputs are evaluated, the process is adjusted to continuously improve it.
6. **Eliminate inappropriate variation.** The sixth step involves implementation. Each specification denotes a measurement point, which is evaluated. One major

goal is to prevent quality failures or variations. Two types of variations will occur. The first is random variation. These variations result from factors inherent in the process, and they occur each time the process is played out. The other form of variation is the specific variation, which is a variation that occurs because of one specific component within the process. Once the processes for improvement are implemented, specific variation frequency should be reduced.

The goal of the CQI process is to eliminate as many specific variations as possible (Deming, 1986). This results in consistently high-quality output.

Within case management, the managed care plans allow for the documentation of variations in clinical practice. By working as a team, the health care professionals can differentiate between random variation and specific variation. The elimination of inappropriate variations results in an approach to health care delivery in which only random variations occur.

Random variations are inherent within every process because every patient is different, and every response to treatment is slightly different. These "noises" in the system occur for every process and affect every output.

7. **Document continuous improvement.** This is the final process and the one that makes continuous improvement possible. Once the opportunities for specific or nonrandom variations have been reduced or eliminated, improvements or innovations are introduced.

Team members can make changes that result in improved quality or increased productivity. Because the opportunity for variation has been reduced, it is easier to evaluate the impact of the innovation. After such evaluation the change either becomes permanent, or the team discontinues its use.

Walter A. Shewhart described this method of using a stable process to test innovations as the *Plan-Do-Check-Act Cycle* (PDCA) (Deming, 1986). First developed in the 1930s, this process has become known as the Shewhart Cycle. See Figure 18-3 (Deming, 1986).

The PDCA Cycle is applied to the process used in case management for addressing and improving health care delivery for particular patient types. Planning involves the identification of specific clinical areas for improvement. As discussed earlier, these areas are either patients in a specific DRG or nurses in a particular unit chosen to undertake the switch to case management.

The **Plan** step involves determining the best managed care plan. The **Do** step involves implementation of the case management approach. The third step, **Check**, involves the analysis of variances that hinder efficient use of the plan. The effects of such variances can be observed by changes in length of stay, patient satisfaction, staff satisfaction, or costs. In some cases, the plan might need further revisions until these tangible results are noted.

The **Act** step is for modifications, if needed. Minimal case management variances indicate that the plan is usable, and can be adopted at that point as the standard. If the variances are not minimal, then the process begins again with the plan changed, tested, checked, and finally adopted.

The aim of the team is to continuously improve the process. In health care,

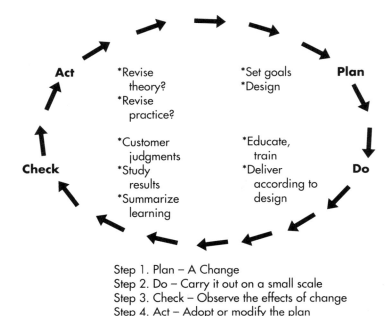

Step 1. Plan – A Change
Step 2. Do – Carry it out on a small scale
Step 3. Check – Observe the effects of change
Step 4. Act – Adopt or modify the plan

Fig. 18-3   The Shewhart Cycle.

the process may never be brought to a conclusion because of the evolutionary nature of the treatment of disease. Changing technology, an aging patient population, and economic considerations, all have a prolonged effect on the delivery of health care. Therefore the process will probably remain open-ended and continuous.

In any case, each process should be seen as one that unremittingly moves forward because today's goals may be tomorrow's standard.

REFERENCES

Berwick, D.M. (1989). Sounding Board. *The New England Journal of Medicine,* January 5, 53-56.

Bryce, G. R. (1991). Quality management theories and their application. *Quality,* February, 23-26.

Crosby, P. B. (1979). *Quality is Free: The Art of Making Quality Certain.* New York: McGraw-Hill.

Deming, W. E. (1986). *Out of the Crisis.* Cambridge: Center for Advanced Engineering Study, Massachusetts Institute of Technology.

Donabedian, A. (1980). *Explorations in Quality Assessment and Monitoring. Vol 1: The Definition of Quality and Approaches to its Assessment.* Ann Arbor, Michigan: Health Administration Press.

Drucker, P. (1991). The new productivity challenge. *Harvard Business Review,* November-December, 67-79.

Goldfield, N. & Nash, D.B. (Eds.) (1989). *Providing quality care.* Philadelphia: American College of Physicians.

Hickman, C. R., & Silva, M. A. (1984). *Creating Excellence: Managing Corporate Culture, Strategy, and Change.* Ontario, NY: New American Library.

Hospital Peer Review. (1988). Deming's Philosophy improves quality. 13(10), 12-24.

Hospitals. (1991). New JCAHO Standards Emphasize Continuous Quality Improvement. August 5, 41-44.

Joint Commission on Accreditation of Hospitals. (1990). *Quality Assessment and Improvement Proposed Revised Standards*. Chicago: The Commission.

Juran, J. M. (1987). *Juran on Quality Leadership: How to go From Here to There*. Wilton, Ct: Juran Institute.

Juran, J. M. (1988). *Juran on Planning for Quality*. New York: Free Press.

Kanter, R.M. (1983). *The change masters: Innovations for productivity in the American Corporation*. New York: Simon & Shuster.

Laffel, G. & Blumenthal, D. (1989). The case for using industrial quality management science in health care organizations. *Journal of the American Medical Association*, Vol. 262(20), 2869-2873.

Marszalek-Gaucher, E. & Coffey, R.J. (1990). *Transforming Healthcare Organizations*. San Francisco, Jossey-Bass.

Naisbitt, J. (1982). *Megatrends: Ten new directions transforming our lives*. New York: Warner Books.

Naisbitt, J., & Aburdene, P. (1985). *Reinventing the Corporation*. New York; Warner Books.

O'Connor, P. (1984). Healthcare financing policy: Impact on nursing. *Nursing Administration Quarterly*, 8(4):10-20.

Quest for Quality and Productivity in Health Services (Sept., 1989). Excerpts from the 1989 Conference Proceedings. Washington, D.C.

Tichy, N. M. & Devanna, M. A. (1986). The transformational leader. *Training and Development Journal*, July, 27-32.

19

Job Satisfaction

CHAPTER OVERVIEW

Many variables affect job satisfaction in the workplace. Among these variables, autonomy, professional status, and socialization are consistently and positively related to increases in satisfaction for registered nurses. Job satisfaction has also been positively related to retention of nurses.

Case management models integrate many of the elements associated with greater job satisfaction, including autonomy, a feeling of connectedness on the job, and professional status.

Two case studies show the relationship between a case management model and job satisfaction. The Nursing Initiatives Program at Long Island Jewish Medical Center in New York demonstrated that the introduction of the case manager role on three pilot units resulted in increased job satisfaction and reduced vacancy rates for registered nurses.

This study was replicated at Beth Israel Medical Center in New York City. Data on three pilot units were collected before start-up and at 9 months. Outcomes demonstrated improved job satisfaction for staff registered nurses and case managers and reductions in vacancy and turnover rates.

JOB SATISFACTION AS A VARIABLE

Among the variables affected by the implementation of a case management model is staff job satisfaction. The introduction of a case manager to a nursing unit can result in an enhanced work environment, which can have a direct effect on the job satisfaction of nurses working there.

The case manager plans and organizes the care of patients who have the most complex cases, assists with patient teaching, and follows through with discharge planning. In an era when many nurses complain that they spend more time documenting patient care, meeting regulatory documentation requirements, filling out requisitions, or making telephone calls than they do with patients, this model provides nurses an opportunity to remain at the bedside while ensuring that all peripheral patient needs are met. Because the case manager relieves staff nurses of some of the indirect nursing functions related to their patients' care, many staff nurses report that they are able to spend more time in direct contact with their patients.

156

Clearly, the case management model builds in a support system to assist busy practitioners in meeting complex patient needs. The model promotes independent practice in those nurses providing the direct patient care. But it does not expect these same nurses to function in a vacuum without the proper support systems to meet all their patients' needs in a rapid-paced and complicated health care environment.

A feeling of job satisfaction has been related to nurse job-turnover rates (Curry, Wakefield, Price, et al, 1985; Reich, 1984; Slavitt, Stamps, Piedmont & Haase, 1978). Choi, Jameson, Brekke, Anderson, and Podratz (1989) demonstrated that nurses' overall dissatisfaction with their work was the strongest predictor of intent to leave the place of employment or current position. Job satisfaction has been directly related to nurse retention and turnover (Hinshaw & Atwood, 1982; Weisman, Alexander & Chase, 1981). Therefore the importance of this variable should not be overlooked when a new nursing-delivery system is being designed or evaluated.

A case management model has an effect on both the staff nurses providing direct patient care and the case managers. The model takes a team approach to care. The team consists of the patient, the family, the physician, the case manager, the direct nursing care provider, the social worker, and others as needed. The model serves to bring all members of the team together with a common focus. Whereas primary nursing led to feelings of isolation and separation for the direct care providers, the case management model does just the opposite. The model's structure works to bring everyone together. Each member supplies information relevant to the care of the patient, and value is placed on every member's input.

As a highly socialized model, case management allows for combined work units organized around a common goal: good patient care. Communication and conflict resolution become needed skills for each team member. If the members of the team cannot function as a group, then the outcomes of care will not be achieved in a timely and efficient manner. Because these are among the primary goals of case management, group dynamics play a significant part in the success or failure of the model.

The case manager role, which fosters teamwork, also provides the nurse with an autonomous job that requires independent thought and action. The support provided by the case manager to the other nurse providers reinforces similar feelings of autonomy and independence in them (Alexander, Weisman & Chase, 1982). It does this by positioning the direct-care provider in a strategic position. A team must rely on the information provided by each of its members, and it is the nurse responsible for direct patient care who provides the information that determines the clinical course of treatment, the teaching needs, and the discharge plan.

This enhanced role for nurses builds feelings of professionalism and self-esteem because nursing's input is valued and deemed important to the patient's progress. In the past, communication was of a hierarchial nature, with the physician dictating to the other members. In the case management model, the nurse case manager serves as the thread that links all members of the team. Each member's input is needed so that appropriate and timely outcomes of care are achieved. In this system, the staff nurse providing direct care at the bedside supplies the case manager and the rest of the team with valuable information.

As discussed in Chapter 22, clinical career ladders help organizations reward both experience and education. A case manager position allows clinically expert, educated, and experienced nurses to take on a role of increasing responsibility while remaining close to the patient. The position provides for a new set of job responsibilities and a new wage scale that takes into account all these factors.

The case management model incorporates those elements that have been correlated to increased job satisfaction and decreased turnover. These elements include autonomy, a feeling of connectedness on the job, and salary (Johnston, 1991; McCloskey, 1990; Pooyan, Eberhardt & Szigeti, 1990).

Some institutions have attempted to measure the satisfaction of their nurses when implementing a case management tool. While it may be said that other factors can affect the nurses' feelings of satisfaction or dissatisfaction with their work—such as the physical work environment, the presence of a computerized clinical information system, the hours of work, or the fringe benefits—some of these other variables can be controlled by testing the same nurses before and after implementation.

CASE STUDIES

In 1988 as part of the United Hospital Fund's Nursing Initiatives Program, five hospitals—The Brooklyn Hospital Center, Long Island Jewish Medical Center, The Neurological Institute of the Presbyterian Hospital, The New York Hospital, and New York University Medical Center—were selected to orchestrate innovative methods for addressing the nursing shortage. Four of the sites proposed and tested new methods of structuring nursing care providers' work, with the goals of increasing nursing productivity, satisfaction, and retention. The fifth site, New York University Medical Center, introduced a stress reduction program with similar goals (Gould & Mezey, 1991).

Long Island Jewish Medical Center, Long Island, New York

At Long Island Jewish Medical Center a new nursing position was created as part of the United Hospital Fund's program. The new position was titled Patient Care Manager and became part of a case management delivery model. The position was specifically designed to match the nurse's expertise with the patient's needs and severity levels. One of the reasons for the new position was to keep nurses at the bedside. The position provided the patient care manager with a challenging and rewarding role (Gould and Mezey, 1991).

Three data collection points were used to gauge nurses' job satisfaction. The first point was before implementation, the second at 1 year, and the third at about 18 months into the project. Job satisfaction was measured by the Nursing Job Satisfaction Scale (Atwood and Hinshaw, 1981; Atwood and Hinshaw, 1984). The instrument, which has been tested for validity and reliability, was given to all nurses on all shifts at each collection point (Ake, Bowar-Ferris, Cesta, et al, 1991).

The medical center's implementation strategies were the following:

- Selecting expert registered nurses as patient care managers
- Assigning patient care managers to coordinate care
- Decentralizing unit decision-making to registered nurses and physicians
- Upgrading nursing-attendant tasks
- Establishing walking rounds

In addition to tracking nurse job satisfaction, registered nurse vacancy rates and registered nurse hours per patient were also evaluated.

Nurses were chosen as patient care managers based on their clinical expertise and willingness to participate in what was, at that time, considered an experimental role.

The three units participating in the project were a 39-bed medical unit, a 32-bed surgical unit, and a 40-bed neonatal intensive care unit (NICU). At the end of the first 18 months of implementation, 20% of the registered nurses on each unit involved were patient care managers. They managed the care provided for one to three patients in addition to their regular direct care functions.

After about 1 year, the patient care managers on the medical unit reported that this dual role was too difficult and stressful. At that time, one patient care manager was recruited to take on the role full time and was removed from direct nursing-role functions. This individual functioned in a truly autonomous and independent case management role.

Average nursing hours per patient remained relatively consistent throughout the project. However, the number of registered nurse hours per patient and the number of registered nurses on the unit decreased from 119.8 FTEs at the start to 113.7 FTEs at 18 months, indicating an increase in productivity.

The registered nurse vacancy rate also improved during the 18-month period. On the medical unit the rate decreased from 8% to 0%, on the surgical unit the vacancy rate decreased from 23% to 0%, and in the NICU it remained constant at 0%.

Among the most dramatic findings was the improvement in nursing job satisfaction, particularly comparing start-up scores to those at 18 months for nurses functioning as patient care managers and those working as staff nurses on the units (See Table 19-1).

Beth Israel Medical Center, New York, New York

The findings of the Nursing Initiatives Program at Long Island Jewish Medical Center pointed to a relationship between nurse roles and responsibilities and job satisfaction. The study was replicated at Beth Israel Medical Center in New York City to determine if the case manager role did indeed play an important part in the job satisfaction of registered nurses.

At the time of implementation of the three pilot units at the Beth Israel Medical Center in January of 1991, all patient care managers were employed on a full-

Table 19-1   Registered nurse satisfaction by service and by title on participating units at Long Island Jewish Medical Center 1988-1990

	At start-up (1988)		At 12 months (1989)		At 18 months (1990)	
	N	Average score	N	Average score	N	Average Score
Service						
Medicine	20	87	26	90	19	94
Surgery	13	92	16	98	15	97
NICU	79	103	69	105	59	105
Total	**112**		**111**		**93**	
Staff PCMs	26	99	17	104	15	110*
Other RNs	86	99	94	100	78	100
Total	**112**		**111**		**93**	

PCMs include all full-time and part-time patient care managers.
*p = .008
Lowest possible score: 23
Highest possible score: 115
(Gould & Mezey, 1991)

Table 19-2   Registered nurse satisfaction by unit and by title on case managed pilot units at Beth Israel Medical Center New York, New York

	At start-up (12/90)		At 9 months (9/91)	
	N	Average score	N	Average score
Unit				
Neurosurgery	11	82	11	82
AIDS	9	88	9	91
Medical-surgical with chemical dependency	10	84	10	90
Total	**30**		**30**	

(T = 2.57, df = 29, p = 0.0157)
Lowest possible score: 23
Highest possible score: 115

time basis, carrying a case load of 15 to 20 patients. Three pilot units were chosen for the study. These units included a 38-bed neurosurgical unit, a 12-bed AIDS unit, and a 45-bed medical/surgical unit for the chemically dependent. One case manager was employed on each unit on a full-time basis, meaning that all three were removed from direct care responsibilities.

Indirect care responsibilities included coordination and facilitation of services to the patient, multidisciplinary care planning, patient and family teaching, and discharge planning.

It was anticipated that the introduction of a case managment model would increase employee job satisfaction. The case managers, working as staff nurses, remained close to the bedside. Relieved of any management responsibilities or

Table 19-3   Patient care managers vs. other registered nurses with data
at both points

	At start-up (12/90)		At 9 months (9/91)	
	N	Average score	N	Average score
Patient care managers	3	78	3	86
Other RNs	27	84	27	89
Total	**30**		**30**	

Not significant at the .05 level.
Lowest possible score: 23
Highest possible score: 115

Table 19-4   Neurosurgery registered nurse vacancy and turnover rates

Time	Vacancy rate	Turnover rate
Start-up	17.33%	21%
9 Months	6%	12.5%

Table 19-5   AIDS unit registered nurse vacancy and turnover rates

Time	Vacancy rate	Turnover rate
Start-up	11%	9%
9 Months	7%	7%

Table 19-6   Medical/surgical unit for chemical dependency registered
nurse vacancy and turnover rates

Time	Vacancy rate	Turnover rate
Start-up	9%	17.6%
9 Months	0%	12%

direct nursing functions, the case managers were not only more easily able to
provide indirect care to the patients, but also to assist other staff nurses.

The case manager was the only staff nurse working a 5-day-a-week schedule.
The case manager was able to fill the information gaps caused by flex-time schedules, which were resulting in fragmented care. This built-in continuity factor
allowed the staff nurse to spend more time in direct patient contact, rather than
reviewing reports or trying to catch up on what happened to the patient in the
nurse's absence.

It was also hypothesized that the introduction of a case management documentation system would enhance registered nurse job satisfaction. The new system, involving the use of MAPs, provided a framework for the nurse to anticipate
care needs on a daily basis. In addition, nursing documentation was collapsed
onto the form itself, eliminating the need for long, narrative notes. Instead of
paragraph notation, the nurse responded to a series of implementation strategies

designed to achieve the goals outlined on the plan. Each 24-hour period was attended to separately, and enough room was provided so that all nurses caring for the patient within that period could document patient progress and outcomes.

The management of patient care provides a structure that addressed length of stay as well as quality of care. Because the case manager is not geographically bound within the nursing unit, this person is the primary caretaker for the patient and family from admission to discharge from the unit. The case manager's lack of geographic constraints and the 5-day-a-week schedule provide for continuity of care for the patient and family.

The case management system, which allows for improved communication between staff members, leads to a greater feeling of teamwork and collegiality. In addition, the enhanced information base from which nurses function provides a greater level of autonomy in their practices.

All registered nurses working on the pilot units were tested for job satisfaction via the Nursing Job Satisfaction Scale (Atwood & Hinshaw, 1981, 1984). Testing took place before implementation and about 9 months after implementation of the case management model. Thirty registered nurses, or 70% of all nurses filling out questionnaires, completed the questionnaire at both data collection points. Of those 30, three were case managers and 27 were staff nurses. All three shifts were represented in the sample.

Job satisfaction scores before start-up and after nine months indicate that there was a statistically significant increase in satisfaction for those nurses working on case managed care units who were there for both data collection periods (See Table 19-2). Comparisons of case managers to other staff nurses at both collection points indicated an increase for both groups (Table 19-3).

For all three units, both registered nurse vacancy rates and turnover rates decreased over the period of the pilot project (See Tables 19-4, 19-5, and 19-6).

On neurosurgery the vacancy rate decreased from 17.33% at startup to 6% at the end of 9 months. The turnover rate decreased from 21% to 12.5%. On the AIDS unit the vacancy rate went from 11% at startup to 7% at the end of 9 months and the turnover rate went from 9% to 7%. The medical/surgical unit for chemically dependent patients achieved a reduction in the vacancy rate from 9% to 0% and a drop in turnover from 17% to 12% at the end of 9 months.

REFERENCES

Ake, J.M., Bowar-Ferris, S., Cesta, T., Gould, D., Greenfield, J., Hayes, P., Maislin, G., and Mezey M. (1991). The nursing initiatives program: Practice based models for care in hospitals. In *Differentiating Nursing Practice: Into the Twenty-First Century*. Kansas City: American Academy of Nursing.

Alexander, C.S., Weisman, C.S., & Chase, G.A. (1982). Determinant's of staff nurses' perceptions of autonomy within different clinical contexts. *Nursing Research, 31*(1), 48-52.

Atwood, J., & Hinshaw, A. (1981). Job Stress: Instrument development program results. *Western Journal of Nursing Research*, 3(3), 48.

Atwood, J., & Hinshaw, A. (1984). Nursing job satisfaction: A program of development and testing. *Research in Nursing and Health*.

Choi, T., Jameson, H., Brekke, M.L., Anderson, J.G., & Podratz, R.O. (1989). Schedule-related effects on nurse retention. Western Journal of Nursing Research, 11(1):92-107.

Curry, J., Wakefield, D., Price, J., Mueller, C., & McCloskey, J. (1985). Determinants of turnover among nursing department employees. *Research in Nursing and Health, 8,* 397-411.

Gould, D.A., & Mezey, M.D. (1991). *At the Bedside: Innovations in Hospital Nursing.* New York: The United Hospital Fund of New York.

Hinshaw, A.S., & Atwood, J.R. (1982). Anticipated turnover: A preventive approach. *Western Journal of Nursing Research, 4,* 54-55.

Johnston, C.L. (1991). Sources of work satisfaction/dissatisfaction for hospital registered nurses. *Western Journal of Nursing Research, 13*(4), 503-513.

McCloskey, J.C. (1990). Two requirements for job contentment: Autonomy and social integration. *Image, 22*(3), 140-143.

Pooyan, A., Eberhardt, B., & Szigeti, E. (1990). Work-related variables and turnover intention among registered nurses. *Nursing and Health Care, 11*(5), 255-258.

Reich, P.A. (1984). *The Relationship Between Jungian Personality Type and Choice of Functional Specialty in Nursing.* Unpublished master's thesis. Adelphi University, Garden City, N.Y.

Slavitt, D.B., Stamps, P.L., Piedmont, E.B., & Haase, A.M. (1978). Nurses satisfaction with their work situation. *Nursing Research, 27,* 114-120.

Weisman, C.S., Alexander, C.S., & Chase, G.A. (1981). Determinants of hospital staff nurse turnover. *Medical Care, 19,* 431-443.

20

Measuring Cost-Effectiveness

CHAPTER OVERVIEW

Measuring cost-effectiveness is one of the most important tasks when evaluating nursing case management models. This chapter reviews a variety of strategies for measuring cost savings in a case management system and provides examples of case studies using these approaches. In addition, suggestions for using these methods in further research are reviewed.

THE EFFECT OF CASE MANAGEMENT ON VARIANCES OF LENGTH OF STAY AND RESOURCE UTILIZATION

In a study done by the American Hospital Association titled *1990 Report of the Hospital Nursing Personnel Survey* (AHA, 1990), the case management model represented the largest increase of nursing care delivery systems most frequently used in the acute care setting. In light of this study and others, it is important to present both current and new methods of evaluating the cost-effectiveness of nursing case management.

In general, case management has been associated with reduced total costs per patient case, decreased patient length of hospital stay, increased patient turnover, and potential increase in hospital-generated revenues.

In a program instituted at Long Regional Hospital in Utah, cost savings were achieved through the use of a bedside-centered case management model (Bair, Griswold & Head, 1989). This approach placed emphasis on the registered nurse to control the use of patient care resources, guide the outcomes of this care within acute care and community-based settings, and, as a member of a multidisciplinary care coordination team, monitor and evaluate the costs and quality components of hospitalization for patients within defined DRG categories.

The registered nurse was given the responsibility and accountability to assess both the inpatient and discharge care requirements and to develop and implement the plan of care related to the prescribed length of stay and amount of patient care resources used. To determine actual costs, focus was placed on the clinical management of defined groups of patients within 10 DRGs or service lines. Each of these groups was analyzed with special emphasis placed on the following areas: patient care services, length of hospitalization, treatment and educational outcomes, discharge and postdischarge care planning, and outpatient and community-based services. Some of the DRGs that were investigated included major joint procedures, angina, heart failure, chest pain, circulatory disorders, acute myocardial infarction, and pneumonia.

A cost containment study, which focused on reducing the average loss per DRG case type, was implemented. A comparison was made of the actual cost per case and the average reimbursement for 10 DRGs. It was demonstrated that bedside case management resulted in cost savings associated with a decrease in length of stay of 0.4 days, an average hospital savings of $284 per case and overall cost savings of $94,572.

Additional savings were realized through strategic planning and better use of patient care resources as evidenced by a reduction in admissions to the intensive care unit by .07 days, and through the accurate assessment and classification of Medicare reimbursement criteria related to inpatient and outpatient group status.

An investigation done by McKenzie, Torkelson, and Holt (1989) showed that interventions associated with nursing case management had a significant effect on patient resource consumption and expenditures.

Case management plans and critical paths were developed for specific high-volume DRGs associated with diseases and disorders of the circulatory system, coronary artery bypass, and catheterization. This study demonstrated average cost savings per case equivalent to $350 for laboratory charges, $180 for radiology charges, and $766 for pharmaceutical charges for nursing case-managed patients. The average length of stay was also reduced by 1.1 days. Within a 1-year period, close to $1 million were saved by using the case management system of care.

Stillwaggon (1989) demonstrated the effect of a nurse model on the cost of nursing care and staff satisfaction. This study was conducted at Saint Francis Hospital and Medical Center in Hartford, Connecticut. An approach to the delivery of patient care called Managed Nursing Care was developed and implemented. This model promoted collaborative practice arrangements, encouraged care based on individualized patient assessment and need, eliminated routine and nonnursing tasks, and established nursing practice guided by professional standards of care. In addition, the professional nurse was able to contract for services and care needed by the patient. This contracting eliminated the need for the traditional work schedule.

The study sample consisted of 100 cases of normal, spontaneous delivery without complication or comorbidity. Comparisons were made between the traditional nursing care delivery system and the new approach to patient care under the nurse managed care model. An assessment was made of the nursing care hours actually delivered and the staff's satisfaction with the nurse managed care model.

Results showed a reduction of 5 hours spent delivering nursing services and a $61.71-decrease in cost of care per case. Additional findings indicated a high level of nursing staff and patient satisfaction with the nurse managed care delivery system.

In another study, Cohen (1991) incorporated a cost-accounting methodology with a combined team nursing/case management model to investigate personnel factors and variable cost components, such as pharmaceuticals and supplies under the nursing case management model. The purpose of this study was to substantiate the financial benefit of using the nursing case management model within the acute care setting.

It was predicted that cesarean section patients who received care under the nursing case management model would have a shorter length of stay than those patients who received care under the existing practices. It was also predicted that the nursing case management system of care would result in an overall decrease in hospital costs and expenditures associated with the cesarean section patient (Cohen, 1991).

The study used a quasi-experimental design on the experimental and control units. The cesarean section case types, DRGs 370 and 371, were selected for study because of the high volume and long length of stay associated with these DRGs. The study sample consisted of 128 cesarean section patients who made up 768 total patient days in 1988. A nonrandom selection was used.

Because randomization was not used, homogeneity controlled for individual extraneous variables that may have affected patient length of stay. Restricting the patient sample to cesarean section helped to control for patient gender, type of diagnosis, and surgical operation.

The data needed for the study required the development and implementation of the nursing case management delivery system. Use of the case management model required thorough orientation for the nursing staff. This orientation period introduced nurses in the experimental group to care under a case management model and helped the case managers assume their roles. Those who were in the experimental group included registered nurses, licensed practical nurses, and nursing assistants. Critical paths and nursing case management care plans were also used.

Demographic data, length of stay, and comorbidity information was received and compiled from the patient subject group. An evaluation was made of professional staff mix as well as the amount of time spent by nurses in delivering patient care (Cohen, 1990; Cohen 1991).

Nursing staff members were expected to cooperate with the investigator of this hospital-based administrative research project. The implementation of the nursing case management model included the following guidelines:

1. The case manager (registered nurse) was responsible for the patient upon admission to the unit.
2. Case associates (co-case managers or primary registered nurses) and case assistants (licensed practical nurses and nursing assistants) were given responsibility for ensuring continuity of care and accountability throughout the patient's length of stay. Each of the co-case managers were assigned different schedules to avoid overlapping days on the unit. Each patient was designated one case manager whose case load was covered by the co-case manager on the case manager's days off.
3. Each case manager was to collaborate with the attending physician in assessing

and evaluating the outcomes of patient care and individualizing the case management plan and critical path.

4. Each case manager was trained to use the case management care plan and critical path to facilitate patient care.
5. The critical path was used for the change-of-shift report.
6. Variance from the case management care plan, the critical path, or both required discussion with the attending physician and a nursing case management consultant.
7. The nursing case manager and physician were to communicate at least twice during the patient's length of stay.
8. The nurse case manager and the patient care coordinator (head nurse) were to collaborate on a daily basis to negotiate assignment planning that would optimize the use of nursing resources.
9. Daily documentation was to reflect the monitoring of patient progress and evaluation of outcomes specified in the case management care plan, variances on the critical path, or both (Cohen, 1990).

COST ACCOUNTING METHOD

One of the primary objectives of the nursing case management system is to develop a cost management information system that validates the patient's use of clinical resources and services and confirms the financial benefits of case management to the institution. In this investigative project, a nursing case management concept was established with the cesarean section case type, which incorporated the following fiscal priorities:

- To maximize control over patient hospital stay by implementing definable and attainable patient goals within a short period of time.
- To decrease service-related costs and enhance DRG reimbursement by reducing patient length of stay through anticipatory planning, early intervention, and the coordination and arrangement of services.

The cost accounting process used in this study involved the four procedural steps described below.

Step I—Establishment of a Resource Use Profile on the Typical Cesarean Section Patient. A historical patient profile that was reflective of conventional practice patterns was developed from the hospital's management information system. This procedure involved a review of detailed charges based on the hospital's charge description and general ledger code reports. These charges were summarized and then compressed from 272 service codes into 14 major clinical use and expense categories. Those categories were then separated by sample group. The categories included routine care, delivery room, operating room, anesthesia, recovery room, laboratory/blood, radiology, respiratory/physiology, general pharmacy, antibiotics, IV (intravenous therapy), other pharmacy, routine treatment, and other.

A two-month sample from 1988 medical records and bills was accessed so that clinical information, financial data, volume of tests and services, posted charge rates for room and board, and ancillary services could be analyzed. An average of the accumulated costs was obtained to arrive at the cost of a unit of service (i.e., patient day, tests, procedures, pharmaceuticals) for all clinically related resources used.

Step II—Establishment of a Resource Use Profile for the Cesarean Section Patient Based on the Nursing Case Management Concept. The historical data obtained from the patient profile were used to develop a patient profile adjusted for nursing case management outcome standards. The major nursing, medical, and ancillary outcome indicators of care were derived from the cesarean section patient's critical path and were used to assess the nursing case management model's efficacy and productivity. Cost standards were set by reducing patient length of stay by 2 days (from 6 to 4 days), streamlining tests and procedures, and initiating patient teaching early in the hospital stay.

Step III—Comparison of the Charge and Resource Use Associated with Comparable Cesarean Section Cases. A charge and clinical resource use comparison was made between the experimental (case management) and control (conventional practice) groups. The comparison involved correlating the average unit of service for both the experimental and control groups to establish the average clinical resource use for the cesarean section patient. For example, the following was identified: average number of tests incurred, average number of supplies used, average number of pharmaceuticals given, average number of nursing care hours provided, and average length of stay. This comparison established a mechanism to monitor the change in resource use after switching from conventional practices to case management. Such monitoring helped ensure that efficient use of services was maintained. The results of this comparison substantiated the efficacy of the case management model.

Step IV—Determination of the Total Average Cost for the Nursing Case Management Model. The above analysis provided the total room and board charges. However, to more effectively determine the average cost of the nursing case management model as well as the required nursing care resources, the following methodology was used: (1) The total direct nursing care costs were computed for both sample groups; (2) nursing care was segregated from total room and board costs; and (3) the ratio of cost to charge (RCC) factor was applied. The comparisons in step III were then categorized by skill mix to determine the number of direct nursing-care hours required under each system for the care of the cesarean section patient.

To determine the total direct nursing-care costs associated with both the experimental and control groups, the following computation was completed:

Average base salary per skill mix by sample group ÷ 1,950 hours (the number of hours worked in a year by an employee) = Average Hourly Wage Rate.

Average hourly wage rate × Sum total of direct nursing care hours provided by skill mix (from the Nursing Case Management Activity Form) × 1.25 (Average Fringe Benefits) = Total average costs of direct nursing care for the cesarean section patient.

The direct nursing care costs were then segregated from the total expenditures to arrive at the remaining room and board costs.

The method used for determining costs was the departmental ratio of cost to charges (RCC), which is the cost-accounting methodology most widely used by health care institutions. The RCC is delineated from the Institutional Cost Report, which is a cost statement used by the Medicare program for various reimbursement processes. This report contains revenue, cost, and clinical service use information by department.

The method involved taking the RCC for each major clinical use and expense category and applying it against the total charges to arrive at an approximate determination of the total cost per case. This provided the final pieces of data needed to establish the total average costs for the nursing case management model (Cohen, 1990; Cohen, 1991).

Findings indicated that a significant reduction in patient length of stay was achieved. Length of stay declined by 1.16 days, or 19%, between the experimental and control groups ($p \leq .0001$). Expenditure and cost analysis showed an increase in direct patient-centered nursing care hours and intensification in use of inpatient services and treatments. This intensification of nursing time and resource use led to the reduction in patient length of stay and a decrease in total overall costs.

The analysis further demonstrated a savings of $930.40 per patient case and a general decrease in hospital costs and expenditures associated with the cesarean section patient. This profit was made possible because of the increase in patient turnover and the availability of additional patient beds. Potential savings and revenues of more than $1 million were identified for the hospital (Cohen, 1991; Health Care Advisory Board, 1990).

Although an analysis of the demographic data showed comparability between the experimental and control groups, the rigor of this investigation can be strengthened by using matched sampling to decrease the likelihood of extraneous variance and by using randomized assignment of the sample groups.

At Beth Israel Medical Center in New York City, the case management model is used as a vehicle for reducing patient length of stay. Coupled with other initiatives such as CQI, reductions in the length of stay for selected diagnoses were realized within the first year of implementing the case management model (See Table 20-1).

Nursing, medicine, social work, administration, patient representatives, operations, and finance were among the departments that participated in the change to a case management delivery system. In some cases, specific medical or surgical departments or specialties were targeted for the development of MAPs. These plans incorporated all professional disciplines in management of the patient's care and ensured outcome-related quality services. In other cases, specific

Table 20-1 Beth Israel Medical Center case managed incremental revenue for selected diagnoses

Diagnosis		DRG(S)	ALOS 1990*
Laminectomy		4/755/756/577 758/214/215	10.0
Endocarditis		126	14.4
Soft tissue infection		278	9.1
Pneumonia		89	11.06
			1/91-6/91
Orthopedics		209/211/233/ 234/218/ 219/220/ 221/223/224	9.0
Diabetes team	Principal diagnosis	294/295/296/ 297/566	9.9
	Secondary diagnosis	—	11.8
	High-risk obstetrics	383	—

diagnoses or DRGs were targeted for significant reductions in length of stay (See Table 20-1).

The Paretto Chart, a statistical tool that can be used to determine which diagnoses or procedures to target, was used for the development of managed care plans and financial analysis (See Fig. 20-1). If an annual review is being conducted, the number of cases for the top volume DRGs can be tallied. These are then placed on the chart in the form of a bar graph in descending order. On the right side of the chart, the percentage of the total cases that each number of cases represents is placed on a cumulative line graph. For example, DRG 707 represented 63 cases, or 31% of the total number of cases. The next highest volume DRG, 277, represented a total of 50 cases, or 24% of the total number of cases. These two percentages are represented cumulatively, as 55% of all cases. This means that these two DRGs represented 55% of all cases admitted to the unit. In most instances, one would study the top 80%, in this case DRGs 707, 277, 708, and 89, which represent approximately 80% of all cases. In this way it is clear that a fair representation of all cases has been included.

Nonunit-based case management teams are committed to following all patients of a specific case type who are admitted to the medical center. They are also responsible for monitoring length of stay, resource use, and quality. The teams also provide in-services to house staff and nursing personnel, to maintain appropriate treatment of these patients.

No. cases 1990	ALOS 1991*	No. cases 1991	Incremental† revenue
260	9.08	213	$ 238,000
94	8.7	58	$ 900,000
189	8.7	156	$ 28,000
298	10.05	257	$ 196,000
1/91-6/91	**7/91-2/92**	**7/91-2/92**	
143	7.08	226	$ 489,000
	11/11/91-1/31/92		
300	3.45	37	
	11/11/91-1/31/92		
—	10.5	29	
—	8.25	12	$ 438,000
		TOTAL	$ 2,289,000

*Length of stay data compiled from an MIS download from the Charms Systems.
†Incremental revenue calculated by Don Modzewleski, Assistant Vice President, Finance.

Two teams, one for diabetes and one for asthma, consisted of several physicians, a nurse case manager, a nurse clinician, and other clinically relevant disciplines. In the case of the diabetes team, a nutritionist was included and functioned as a full-time member who saw all patients assigned to the team.

The managed care plan is used to guide care and to provide a framework for keeping the length of stay in check. The length of stay on the plan is determined by studying the region, state, and federal lengths of stay for those DRGs relevant to the diagnosis or procedure. The physician practice patterns are then reviewed, and length of stay for the institution is established for that diagnosis.

Two groups for case management, unit-based case managers and nonunit-based case managers, were developed. The unit-based case managers assumed the same role as the nonunit-based case manager. However, the unit-based manager's primary responsibility was on an individual unit level and involved more than one diagnosis and many different physicians. The unit-based case manager can be equally effective because that person sees the patient several times during the day, intervening whenever necessary. The nonunit-based case managers, on the other hand, may spend a portion of the day traveling from one unit to another. Therefore their time with each patient is more limited.

Both groups, the nonunit-based case managers and the unit-based case managers, were able to demonstrate significant cost reductions within the first few

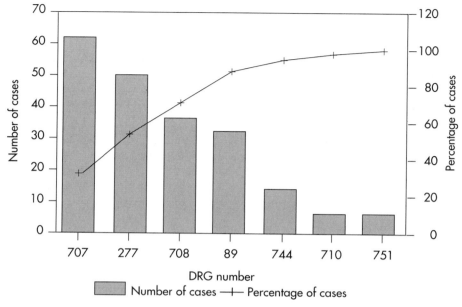

Key:
707 HIV infection with opioid use
227 Cellulitis
708 HIV without opioid use
89 Pneumonia
744 Opioid abuse
710 HIV other
751 Alcohol

Fig. 20-1 1991 DRG Paretto Chart.

weeks and months of implementation. Once the targeted diagnoses had been identified, the institution's prior length of stay history was obtained. These data allowed the team to determine what the expected length of stay would have been if the conventional model of patient care had been used.

After implementation of case management, the length of stay was tracked on a monthly basis for those patients followed by the case management approach. Patients with certain diagnoses or surgical procedures were targeted and followed by the case manager.

Stringent data collection was necessary for accurate cost accounting. Preimplementation length-of-stay data provided the framework for determining whether the length-of-stay goals were achieved.

RELATIVE WEIGHTS AND FINANCIAL ANALYSIS

Some diagnoses fall within a single DRG. For example, "pneumonia" will almost always be coded within DRG 89. Conversely, many surgical procedures can be classified within a number of DRG categories. For example, laminectomy can be coded within as many as seven DRGs. Each of these DRGs may have a different financial weight.

The weights applied to each DRG are called *relative weights*. The relative weight is a value applied to the DRG based on the average complexity and resource consumption for patients within that DRG. The relative weight for "carpal tunnel release" will be much lower than the relative weight for "major chest procedures," which is one of the highest weighted DRGs. The relative weight will apply differently for Medicare versus other third party payers.

Institutions performing a larger number of procedures with higher relative weight values will see a higher overall reimbursement, reflective in the Case Mix Index (CMI) for each department and ultimately the institution. The CMI provides an indication of the relative costliness of providing care and is determined by taking an average of all the service intensity weights over all discharges for the institution. The service intensity weights are the average of all the weights of all DRGs seen on a particular service.

For example, transplants carry an extremely high relative weight. If an institution performs a large number of transplants, this will inflate the overall CMI, resulting in a greater financial appearance. Complexity and intensity form the basis of the CMI system. Although there is no clear definition of complexity, it generally refers to the types of services rendered, while intensity refers to the number of services per patient day or hospital stay (Luke, 1979).

There is some incentive in this system for health care organizations to bring in larger numbers of patients whose DRG will be of a higher relative weight. This has often resulted in many hospitals offering these types of services with less emphasis on the lower paying groups.

Beth Israel Medical Center used the relative weight values as a basis for determining the financial gain or loss of each of the diagnoses or procedures tracked under the case management system. If the diagnosis being evaluated falls within one DRG, the process is much easier. In the case of endocarditis, the length of stay for case managed patients decreased from 14.4 days in 1990 to 8.7 days in 1991. This length-of-stay reduction was analyzed against the number of cases at the shorter length of stay and the relative weight for the DRG.

A relative cost weight is obtained by dividing the adjusted national cost per DRG by the adjusted national cost per case for all DRGs. The larger the relative cost weight, the greater the relative costliness of a DRG (Grimaldi & Micheletti, 1983).

An assumption was made that for each day's reduction in length of stay, the bed was "back-filled" with a patient falling into a DRG with the same or greater relative weight. In this way, although the length of stay was decreased, available beds were utilized.

In other cases the surgical procedure being analyzed fell under more than one

DRG, as in the case of laminectomies. In this circumstance, the relative weight for all possible DRGs must be averaged.

With case management teams that potentially could be managing several DRGs, the same process would be followed. The average relative weight would be averaged for all possible DRGs, again assuming the beds would be back-filled with similar patients.

Although this type of cost-accounting system is not completely precise, it does give a good indication of the approximate incremental revenue savings for the diagnosis or surgical procedure under analysis.

IMPLICATIONS FOR FURTHER RESEARCH

All the studies reviewed share common implications for clinical and professional practice. One implication is in the area of assessing the quality of the critical path analysis and MAPs. Both the critical path and MAP were used to set clinical resource and cost standards and were responsible for most of the planning, coordination, and integration activities of the nursing case management model. Future research would be helpful for evaluating the critical path's and MAP's reliability and validity. Additional research should also focus on the treatment and practice protocols developed by the critical path and MAP analysis as they relate to patient care and clinical practice outcomes.

One other major implication is in objectively measuring the contributions of the nursing case management model to the quality of patient care, in particular, its effects on patient care resources, and in assessing patient and provider satisfaction. Additional research is needed to look at the effects of nursing case management on professional autonomy and decision-making opportunities for nurses, collaborative practice arrangments between nurses and physicians, nursing case management staffing and assignment allocations, payment and reimbursement mechanisms for nursing case management services, and the types of nursing case management interventions used and the effects of these interventions on patient outcomes. Other general implications for nursing follow:

- The changes in practice patterns associated with nursing case management can help to reduce overall expenditures related to hospitalization.
- Nursing case management can provide substantial improvements in the cost-effectiveness of patient care.
- Nursing case management focuses on collaborative practice arrangements between nurses and physicians to help shorten length of hospital stay and maintain effective use of money and materials thereby having a significant effect on the hospital's fiscal bottom line and viability.
- Nursing case management has the potential to equate the effects of clinical nursing services and outcomes with resource allocation, costs, and reimbursement systems.
- Nursing case management has the potential to positively affect the present nursing care shortage by reorganizing delivery systems to maximize professional decision-making opportunities for nurses and allowing for continuity of patient care.

- Nursing case management can relate the cost savings of nursing interventions to specific patient populations in the acute care setting.
- Nursing case management can enhance the management of nursing services and substantiate the economic accountability and contribution of nurses to consumers of health care services.

Nursing case management provides the baseline for further research and evaluation of the functional competencies and uses of different skill levels in delivering nursing care services to patients and their families. This approach allows for more efficient integration of various levels of support staff by defining role expectations. Cohen's (1990) study successfully used the registered nurse as the case manager and case associate with the nursing assistants as support staff. The nurse case manager coordinated, assessed, evaluated, and participated with the case associates in the delivery of patient care. The nursing assistants carried out tasks associated with the patients' activities of daily living as delegated by the nurse case manager.

REFERENCES

American Hospital Association (1990). *1990 report of the hospital nursing personnel survey.* Chicago: American Hospital Association.

Bair, N., Griswold, J., & Head, J. (1989). Clinical RN involvement in bedside-centered case management. *Nursing Economics, 7*(3), 150-154.

Cohen, E. (1990). *The effects of a nursing case management model on patient length of stay and variables related to cost of care delivery within an acute care setting.* Dissertation Abstracts International, 51-07B, 3325 (University Microfilm No. 90-33878), Ann Arbor, Mich.: University Micro Films International.

Cohen, E. (1991). Nursing case management: Does it pay? *Journal of Nursing Administration, 21*(4), 20-25.

Grimaldi, P.L. & Micheletti, J.A. (1983). *Diagnosis related groups.* Chicago: Pluribus Press.

Health Care Advisory Board (1990). Tactic #1 potential savings of more than $1 million from change in delivery system, use of critical paths for two DRGs. Superlative Clinical Quality: special review of pathbreaking ideas, clinical quality (1) (pp. 23) Washington, D.C.: Advisory Board Co.

Luke, R.D. (1979). Dimensions in hospital case mix measurement. *Inquiry, 16*(Spring), 38-49.

McKenzie, C., Torkelson, N. & Holt, M. (1989). Care and cost: Nursing case management improves both. *Nursing Management, 20*(10), 30-34.

Stillwaggon, C. (1989). The impact of nurse managed care on the cost of nurse practice and nurse satisfaction. *Journal of Nursing Administration, 19*(11), 21-27.

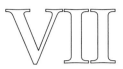

ISSUES FOR CONSIDERATION

21

Organized Labor and Case Management

CHAPTER OVERVIEW

Nursing administrators generally believe that nursing case management models cannot be implemented in unionized facilities. This chapter demonstrates that these two concepts are not mutually exclusive. Nurse administrators in unionized environments can use the strategies discussed in this book to implement case management models in their hospitals. It is also worthwhile to consider organized labor's own interest in containing the costs associated with providing health care for union members. The concepts of nursing case management are of interest to organized labor because the model provides those *in* the union with high-quality, cost-effective care.

CASE MANAGEMENT IN UNIONIZED FACILITIES

For those departments of nursing represented by collective bargaining unions or state associations, special consideration is needed when implementing case management. Initial planning for the model will require determining whether or not the case manager position will be a union or management position. This decision will probably depend on the job description and philosophy of the position.

If the case manager position is one that will be filled by a staff nurse, it would then be rational to leave it within the union. However, if clinical nurse specialists are used as case managers, or if the case manager position is not considered to be an option on the career-ladder, it may then be more appropriate to designate it as a nonunion position.

If the staff nurses of the institution are represented by collective bargaining, leaving the position in the union as a staff level position may result in the forfeiture of some of the position's autonomy. For example, the staff level nurse will be limited by rules and regulations concerning work hours, vacation and holiday time, conference time, and time off the unit. The nature of the case manager job requires the nurse to spend additional periods of time off the unit meeting with

179

other professional disciplines, doing research for the managed care plans, or attending in-service programs. This freedom of movement will be restricted by collective bargaining agreements to which every staff nurse must conform.

On the other hand, removing the position from the bargaining unit may send a negative message that indicates to staff and others that excellence can only be achieved by using someone outside the bargaining unit. Conversely, a management position within a unionized facility will mean more autonomy and independence for the case manager.

If it is decided that the position will remain as a career ladder option within the collective bargaining unit, the union must be included as early as possible in decisions regarding salary, job description, and title.

It is likely that there will be minimal resistance from the union if the position is left within the union. The position will provide opportunities to reward outstanding performance with an internal promotion for staff nurses, resulting in an increase in salary and advanced role. By keeping the case manager position as part of the organized union, there will be no erosion in bargaining power for the unit member. If the organization implementing case management desires a quick implementation period, then making the position part of the union might be the path of least resistance. Philosophically, the message will be made clear. Excellence can occur within the union as well as without, and one does not need to be in a management position to achieve a level of autonomy or accountability.

Negotiations with the union include issues of salary. Other issues to be negotiated should certainly include daytime working hours, rotation, holidays, and weekends. Case managers should be on duty Monday through Friday, when they can have the greatest effect on patient care. It is during these time periods that they are best able to meet with other disciplines, as well as facilitate tests, treatments, or procedures. The transition will be smoother if these issues are negotiated with the union before implementation.

CASE MANAGEMENT: ORGANIZED LABOR'S RESPONSE TO ESCALATING HEALTH CARE COSTS

In discussing the role of organized labor in nursing case management, it may be helpful to consider organized labor's interest in providing high-quality, reasonably priced health care to its own union members.

As health care becomes more expensive, organizations are looking toward case management to assist in managing and controlling spiraling health care costs. Case management and other corporate health care alternatives are being integrated into employees' medical and liability benefit plans, worker's compensation and disability, long-term care and retiree services, and dependent care initiatives (Frieden, 1991b; Katz, 1991). Case management has also been successful in providing and maintaining quality, cost-effective mental health care services, prenatal care, and employee health promotion programs.

Along these lines, labor organizations have also begun to initiate cooperative alliances with management in an effort to contain health care costs (Bell, 1991).

Maintaining health care and insurance benefits has become a priority of union leaders according to a survey conducted by Metropolitan Life (Data Watch, 1991).

A 1991 survey by the Health Research Institute showed a willingness by both labor and management groups to develop health care programs that support early prevention and primary care services (Data Watch, 1991).

Other joint arrangements between labor and management have led to the development of initiatives that offer stress and mental health counseling, substance abuse programs, preemployment screening, child and dependent care support, disability, case management, access to health care service networks, such as on-site medical care, outpatient care, home health care, community-based programs, and health awareness education (Bell, 1991; Beresford, 1991; Chelius, Galvin & Owens, 1992; Jordahl, 1992; Lucas, 1991).

Efforts to maintain employee health-benefit levels while reducing expenses have led some corporations to contract with PPOs (See Chapter 8). These arrangements have helped ensure accessibility and affordability to needed health care services (Ciccotelli, 1991; Varecha, Barry & Martingale, 1991).

Organized labor has also begun to launch national health reform campaigns. These efforts are aimed at implementing a national social health insurance plan, controlling medical service reimbursement, providing universal health care coverage, coordinating and managing administrative activities, and providing access to long-term, community-based health care services (Frieden, 1991a).

Innovative approaches to delivering and maintaining health care services will become more prevalent as the economic environment continues to grow more complex and difficult to manage. Hospitals currently involved in restructuring interests have joined with labor groups to focus efforts on providing quality, cost-effective patient care. This goal has been achieved in some settings with the deployment of nursing case management, both in union and management positions.

REFERENCES

Bell, N. (1991). Workers and managers of the world unite! *Business and Health, 9*(8), 26-34.

Beresford, L. (1991). Union wants a soberer image. *Business and Health, 9*(8), 51-54.

Chelius, J., Galvin, D. & Owens, P. (1992). Disability: It's more expensive than you think. *Health, 11*(4), 78-84.

Ciccotelli, C. (1991). Union engineers a better health care system. *Business and Health, 9*(8), 56-57.

Data Watch: Unions and health care. (1991). *Business and Health, 9*(8), 8-9.

Frieden, J. (1991a). Unions rev up health reform engines. *Business and Health, 9*(8), 42-50.

Frieden, J. (1991b). What's ahead for managed care? *Business and Health, 9*(13), 43-49.

Jordahl, G. (1992). Labor/management partnerships foster better employee relationships. *Business and Health, 9*(4), 73-76.

Katz, F. (1991). Making a case for case management. *Business and Health, 9*(4), 75-77.

Lucas, B. (1991). Armour foods thin slices workers' compensation costs. *Business and Health, 9*(8), 58-60.

Varecha, R., Barry J. & Martingale, J. (1991). Laboring to manage care. *Business and Health, 9*(8), 35-41.

22

Clinical Ladders

CHAPTER OVERVIEW

Nursing career ladders can be intrinsically linked to a case management model. The case manager position can be integrated as the third or fourth rung of a clinical ladder. In this way, the increased experience and education of the more advanced role is rewarded in a bedside position that recognizes and rewards experience. Traditional clinical ladders are often unable to meet both educational and experiential needs of the advanced practitioner. The autonomous case manager role is attractive to nurses with experience who wish to remain in bedside nursing but who are looking for a position of increased responsibility and independent practice.

When considering clinical ladders, institutions need to assess the cost of maintaining a ladder and evaluate the positive effects such a ladder has on recruitment and retention.

GOALS AND OBJECTIVES OF A CAREER LADDER

The nursing case management model can provide the framework for the integration of a true clinical ladder. Traditionally, clinical ladders have not provided a system for promotion at the bedside that included true changes in job title and responsibility.

The majority of promotions at the bedside have provided the staff nurse with an elevated title, such as Staff Nurse Level II or Senior Staff Nurse. This change in title may have also included a financial reward and an altered job description. However, analysis of such positions reveals that the actual day-to-day responsibilities remained the same.

Each organization implementing a career ladder will have different goals and objectives for an addition of this kind. Generally, the integration of a career ladder will cost the organization money. The long-term savings that come because of decreased turnover or lowered vacancy rates are difficult to measure. Even more difficult is showing a cause-and-effect relationship between the career ladder and the decreased turnover and vacancy rates (Vestal, 1984).

Nevertheless, there are some generic goals and objectives that most organizations will hope to achieve by implementing a career ladder. Whether the achievement of these goals offsets the cost of maintaining the increased salaries that accompany the ladder will be a choice each organization must make for itself (Del Bueno, 1982).

The inherent benefits of an effective clinical career ladder include the following:

- Providing the opportunity for professional advancement in a direct patient-care position
- Promoting individual professional growth and development
- Attracting and retaining nurses to the organization
- Providing a mechanism for rewarding individual expertise
- Providing a framework for the development of performance evaluation tools
- Increasing job satisfaction
- Having a positive effect on patient care

Most clinical career ladders reflect what the name suggests. The ladders are designed to promote clinical advancement, usually at the bedside. Therefore the emphasis is on the direct care provider, generally the staff nurse. Other ladders may be designed for career or professional advancement, such as administration or education, or they may be a combination of clinical, administration, and education.

Each step or level must be defined by specific behaviors and levels of performance that are identifiable and measurable. They should also be realistic and achievable (AORN, 1983).

Advancement in the clinical ladder is initiated by the nurse through a request. It is the nurse's responsibility to produce documents supporting a claim for advancement to the next level. Evaluation will then take place through a review of the documents. The documents should include the nurse's periodic evaluations, and any other evidence of professional education, certification, and the like.

The documents are weighed against the performance expectations of the level to which the nurse is striving. Theoretically, any nurse who has met the criteria should be eligible for advancement. In a true career ladder situation, there should be no quota of positions per level, and any qualified nurse should be eligible for the advancement.

All nurses within the career ladder should be evaluated periodically. These evaluations result in advancement, remaining in the current position, or demotion (AORN, 1983).

Incentives for promotion include advanced title, salary benefits, and heightened status. Each promotional level should move the nurse toward a higher level of empowerment and self-actualization.

Just as there are benefits to the implementation of a ladder, there are also some problems (McKay, 1986). As already mentioned, the cost/benefit ratio may not be suitable for the organization. There is always the potential for a ladder to create a negative effect because it implies a hierarchical organizational structure.

For the ladder to result in a truly supportive environment and improved quality of care, staffing patterns for each day and for each shift should incorporate a mixture of representatives from each level. This may not always be feasible or realistic, particularly on the evening or night shift when staffing levels are low.

Monetary awards are often greater for those advancing within an administrative career ladder than those advancing within a clinical ladder.

Other difficulties arise if the nursing department is represented by a union. The goals of the department and the goals of the clinical ladder must meld with those of the union. Each aspect of the ladder needs to be negotiated for integration into the bargaining union contract. Nursing departments represented in this way should include union representatives in the negotiations from the very beginning. In most cases, the institution of a clinical career ladder will be best implemented at the beginning of a new contract.

The number of levels of any ladder will depend upon the philosophy, goals, and budget of the organization. The following is a list of characteristics that a nurse from a particular level should have.

Level I:

- Entry level capabilities
- A license or temporary permit to practice professional nursing
- An understanding of the hospital policies and procedures
- A basic familiarity with patient care
- General skills needed to function at a beginning level of nursing practice

Level II:

- A more holistic understanding of patient care delivery
- A career orientation with goals and direction
- An ability to prioritize needs of patients and families and to delegate responsibilities to other members of the nursing staff as appropriate
- An ability to act as a resource for other nursing staff members
- An understanding of the relationship between career goals and personal growth

Level III:

- Ability to act as a resource for the health care team
- Self-directed in most aspects of learning
- Involvement in professional committees, organizations or both
- An understanding of the health care team as a whole that comes together to meet mutual patient goals
- A change agent for the institution within the department of nursing
- An active seeker of additional professional responsibility
- Commitment to nursing as a career
- Ability to plan patient care based on current and future patient care needs
- Ability to plan for appropriate discharge
- Financial awareness incorporated into daily practice, including resource use, length of stay, and discharge planning needs

The level I registered nurse is expected to apply basic nursing theory to practice. Nursing care is delivered to the nurse's assigned group of patients based on actual needs, physician orders, and nursing diagnoses. The registered nurse at level I is able to complete all required treatments for a particular shift in accordance with the policies and procedures of the organization. This nurse may begin to learn the skills necessary to assess patient and family learning needs and to begin meeting those needs (Barr & Desnoyer, 1988).

The level II practitioner begins to shift from actual patient problems to identifying potential problems and applying interventions that will prevent those problems from occurring. At this level the nurse's organizational skills begin to develop. Focus becomes more global as the nurse develops an awareness of not only the nurse's own patients, but those throughout the unit. Patient problems are seen on a health care continuum that extends beyond hospitalization (Barr & Desnoyer, 1988).

The level III practitioner sees the health care team as a whole and seeks to begin to bring the team together to meet patient needs and to provide the best possible care. At this level the nurse begins to take a more active leadership role on the unit, serving as preceptor and informal leader. The registered nurse at this level is involved in seeking advanced education in some specialty or certification category. The nurse applies this knowledge and skill in practice and becomes an expert in the chosen area. This knowledge is used by the expert nurse to create an environment for positive change both on the unit and in the department (Barr & Desnoyer, 1988).

Differentiated practice is a personnel deployment model designed to better use the skills and education of the experienced nurse. An educational requirement within a clinical performance framework is incorporated into the differentiated practice model. By using a differentiated practice modality, the design of the clinical ladder can clearly delineate the evolving knowledge base and expanded level of functioning of the experienced nurse. Some institutions may want to include criteria for educational level and mandate that those at the third or fourth level have a master's degree. By using this model within a clinical ladder, employee's roles are based on both educational preparation and clinical performance.

In other models, the fourth or fifth level is that of the clinical nurse specialist. If this role is seen as a bedside clinical position and not as a management or educator position, this position belongs in a clinical career ladder. Once again, this depends on the placement of the role within the department (Metcalf, 1984).

THE CASE MANAGER POSITION WITHIN THE CLINICAL LADDER

The case manager position provides the opportunity for the development of a true career ladder, one that integrates a title change and financial incentive with significant changes in job description and job responsibilities.

The staff nurse position incorporates all the direct nursing tasks associated with providing nursing care. Included among these are the physical assessment, vital signs, medication administration, blood-drawing, wound care, skin care, ambulation, and patient feedings.

The generic nurse case manager role removes the staff nurse from direct nursing functions. Her role becomes one concerned with the indirect nursing tasks that are provided to patients. Among these are patient and family teaching, care planning, coordination and facilitation of patient care and services, and discharge planning.

Shifting the focus to these functions also involves a substantial increase in the number of patients that can be taken care of on a daily basis. A case manager's focus is much broader than just the tasks at hand. The case manager must constantly focus on the plan of care for the days ahead by coordinating and facilitating services whether for discharge planning or patient teaching.

For the first time, this group of nurses has been given responsibility for controlling costs and length of stay. In this position, nursing holds the purse strings of health care.

Furthermore, this is the first time, a registered nurse who wishes to remain at the bedside can do so while accepting promotion and change in job status. This position can be very attractive to nurses who are not interested in positions within administration or education, but who are looking for a change that still involves bedside nursing. In other cases, the position might be attractive to a nurse who may have been in the field for 1 or 2 years and does not yet have the skills or education needed to advance to administrative or educational roles.

The case manager position is usually found at the third or fourth level of a clinical career ladder. The position empowers the staff nurse to create an environment for change in the organization, and it has the potential to result in a tremendous amount of job satisfaction. Research shows that longevity and job satisfaction are related (Malik, 1992). The career ladder, therefore, provides an incentive for the more experienced nurse to remain in a clinical position. Increased job satisfaction may have a trickle-down effect on the other staff nurses on the unit.

The autonomous case manager role may be the best argument thus far for creating clinical career ladders. Malik (1992) reports that clinical career ladders may not provide a position that affords the experienced staff nurse the opportunity to use her advanced skills and knowledge. The case manager role, which requires a higher level of functioning and skills, may serve to fill this gap.

REFERENCES

AORN (1983). Guidelines for developing clinical ladders. *AORN Journal, 37*(6), 1209-1224.

Barr, N.J. & Desnoyer, J.M. (1988). Career development for the professional nurse: A working model. *The Journal of Continuing Education in Nursing, 19*(2), 68-72.

Del Bueno, D. (1982). "A clinical ladder? Maybe!". *Journal of Nursing Administration,* September, 19-22.

Malik, D.M. (1992). Job satisfaction related to use of career ladder. *Journal of Nursing Administration, 22*(3), 7.

McKay, J.I. (1986). Career ladders in nursing: An overview. *Journal of Emergency Nursing, 12*(5), 272-278.

Metcalf, J. (1984). The clinical nurse specialist in a clinical career ladder. *Nursing Administration Quarterly,* Fall, 8-19.

Vestal, K.W. (1984). Financial considerations for career ladder programs. *Nursing Administration Quarterly,* Fall, 1-8.

1

BETH ISRAEL MEDICAL CENTER

MULTI-DISCIPLINARY ACTION PLAN

DIAGNOSIS: <u>ASTHMA (PEDIATRICS)</u>

MD: <u>PEDIATRIC AMBULATORY GROUP</u>

UNIT: <u>PEDIATRIC – INPATIENT</u>

ADMISSION DATE: _____

DATE MAP INITIATED: _____

DRG #:   <u>98/774/775</u>

EXPECTED LENGTH OF STAY: <u>4 DAYS</u>

PATIENT CARE MANAGER: _____

SOCIAL WORKER: _____

PATIENT ALLERGIES: _____

YES/NO   DATE

DNR:

Copyright Beth Israel
Medical Center 1992
All rights reserved

HEALTH CARE PROXY

OR LIVING WILL: _____

```
          BETH ISRAEL MEDICAL CENTER
       MULTI-DISCIPLINARY ACTION PLAN

              DAY 1 OF 4


   MD: _____

   DIAGNOSIS: _____

   RN/MD REVIEW: _____
```

DATE: _____

MAP DOES NOT REPLACE MD ORDERS ·   **VARIANCE**

TESTS/ PROCEDURES/ TREATMENTS	CBC, Theophylline level, SMA6, PPD. Initiate chest PT before NEB TX. Dipstick Urine X1, Check specific gravity X1. Ask for old chart & problem face sheet from clinic chart. When indicated order should include: Peak flow >6yrs. or cooperative qshift., ABG'S, CXR, pulse oximeter, postural drainage	
MEDICATIONS	(amt. according to wt. in kg's.) IV Aminophylline and/ or Proventil NEB/PO and/or Steroids (Solucortef, solumedrol, Prednisone and/or Cromolyn and/or Oxygen.)	
ACTIVITY	As tolerated	
NUTRITION	As tolerated	
CONSULTS	None	
SOCIAL WORK		
DISCHARGE PLANNING	Determine if Home Care Services were provided prior to admission. Consult with social worker regarding initial screening and projected discharge plan.	
PATIENT VARIANCE (On Admission)		

DATE	INITIALS	PRINT NAME	SIGNATURE

BETH ISRAEL MEDICAL CENTER
MULTI-DISCIPLINARY ACTION PLAN

DAY 1 OF 4

MD: _____

DIAGNOSIS: _____

DATE: _____

MAP DOES NOT REPLACE MD ORDERS

PATIENT PROBLEM	EXPECTED PATIENT OUTCOME/ DISCHARGE OUTCOME	NURSING INTERVENTIONS		ASSESSMENT/ INTERVENTION
1. Alteration in breathing pattern	1. Pt. will be free of respiratory distress as evidenced by: A. Resp. rate within normal limits for age. B. Arterial blood gases within normal limits. C. Equal air movement heard on auscultation. D. Clear breath sounds. E. Minimal work effort for breathing.	1A. Auscultate breath sounds: Assess adventitious breath sounds (wheezing stridor, rhonchi, rales). B. Assess color changes of skin, mucous membrane, ex: pallor, cyanosis. C. Assess and observe for retractions and nasal flaring q4 hrs, and more frequently during the acute attack. D. Observe for agitation, anxiety. E. Note changes in VS, BP, or O2 saturation if on oximeter. F. Position in manner most comfortable and to facilitate chest expansion. G. Monitor response to tx. (Report to MD resp. distress, vomiting, headache, agitation, tachycardia) H. Chest P/T once per shft, unless otherwise contraindicated. I. Check specific gravity, dipstick urine X one. J. Enc. fluids if tolerating po. K. Peak flow qshift, if child >6yrs. L. Assess pt's. response to activitiy.		
2. Knowledge deficit	2. The parent/child will verb. knowledge of teaching done regarding: A. Precipitating factors (Allergens, smoke, sudden changes in temp.). B. Meds, names, dose desired effects, adverse effects, frequency and times. C. Importance of regular follow-up appointments. D. Exercise regimen with breathing exercises.	2A. Orient to room and unit. B. Assess readiness to learn. C. Familiarize with treatment regimen, i.e. IV pump, Medications, respiratory nebulizer treatment, peak flow meter.		
3. Anxiety	3A. De-escalation of anxiety to within coping levels. B. Identify stress factors.	3A. Provide quiet calm environment, minimize anxiety producing situations. B. Explore stressors and coping mechanisms. C. Assess family dynamics.		

```
      BETH ISRAEL MEDICAL CENTER

   MULTI-DISCIPLINARY ACTION PLAN


           DAY 2 OF 4


  MD: _____

  DIAGNOSIS: _____

  RN/MD REVIEW: _____
```

DATE: _____

MAP DOES NOT REPLACE MD ORDERS   **VARIANCE**

TESTS/ PROCEDURES/ TREATMENTS	Theophylline level, ABG's if indicated. Peak flow every shift if >6yrs "or" cooperative q8 hrs. Chest PT/Postural Drainage	
MEDICATIONS	Steroids could be discontinued within 48 hours or taper over a period of 7-10 days. Assess for change to PO meds.	
ACTIVITY	As tolerated	
NUTRITION	As tolerated	
CONSULTS	None	
SOCIAL WORK	Screen to identify psychosocial and discharge planning needs. Begin social work assessment for hi-risk patients: If patient has been or is being reported to Child Welfare Administration, document all pertinent information, especially registry number.	
DISCHARGE PLANNING	Request Home Health Care evaluation as indicated.	
PATIENT VARIANCE (On Admission)		

DATE	INITIALS	PRINT NAME	SIGNATURE

BETH ISRAEL MEDICAL CENTER
MULTI-DISCIPLINARY ACTION PLAN

DAY 2 OF 4

MD: _____

DIAGNOSIS: _____

DATE: _____

MAP DOES NOT REPLACE MD ORDERS

PATIENT PROBLEM	EXPECTED PATIENT OUTCOME/ DISCHARGE OUTCOME	NURSING INTERVENTIONS	ASSESSMENT/ INTERVENTION	
1. Alteration in breathing pattern	1. Pt. will be free of respiratory distress as evidenced by: A. Resp. rate within normal limits for age. B. Arterial blood gases within normal limits. C. Equal air movement heard on auscultation. D. Clear breath sounds. E. Minimal work effort for breathing.	1A. Auscultate breath sounds: Assess adventitious breath sounds (wheezing, stridor, rhonchi, rales). B. Assess color changes of skin, i.e pallor and cyanosis. C. Assess and observe for retractions and nasal flaring q4 hrs. and more frequently during the D. Note changes in VS, BP, or O2 Saturation (if on oximeter) and readiness to D/C pulse Oximetry. E. Chest P/T once per shift, unless otherwise ordered or contraindicated. F. Monitor response to tx. Report to MD increase resp. distress, vomiting, headache, agitation, tachycardia. G. Peak flow every shift if >6 yrs. H. Assess pt's. response to activity. I. Encourage fluids if tolerating po.		
2. Knowledge deficit	2. The parent/child will verb. knowledge of teaching done regarding: A. Precipitating factors (Allergens, smoke, sudden changes in temp.). B. Meds, names, dose desired effects, adverse effects, frequency and times. C. Importance of regular follow-up appointments. D. Exercise regimen with breathing exercises.	2A. Assess family and patients knowledge base of disease process and begin discharge teaching. B. Assess need for VNS (initiate if applicable). C. Community referrals (ex. N.Y. Lung Assoc.)		
3. Anxiety	3A. De-escalation of anxiety to within coping levels. B. Identify stress factors.	3A. Allow for verbalization of feelings, fears, and anxieties. B. Provide emotional support. C. Reevaluate level of anxiety PRN, provide supportive measures. D. Teach regarding guided imagery, diversional activities.		

BETH ISRAEL MEDICAL CENTER

MULTI-DISCIPLINARY ACTION PLAN

DAY 3 OF 4

MD: _____

DIAGNOSIS: _____

RN/MD REVIEW: _____

DATE: _____

MAP DOES NOT REPLACE MD ORDERS **VARIANCE**

TESTS/ PROCEDURES/ TREATMENTS	Check PPD, Theophylline level Peak flow every shift if >6yrs "or" cooperative q8 hrs. Chest PT/Postural Drainage	
MEDICATIONS	Assess change to po medications i.e. Slobid, Somophyl-line, Proventil, Steroids	
ACTIVITY	As tolerated	
NUTRITION	As tolerated	
CONSULTS		
SOCIAL WORK	Continue involvement in discharge planning; ongoing consultation with patient, family, MD, RN, and HHIC. On the day prior to discharge: Finalize D/C plan, verify-parent/caregiver avail., clothing, etc. Confirm trans., home care plans with HHIC & CCMU as needed. Coordinate prep. of req. documents for trans. e.g. inter-institutional transfer form etc.	
DISCHARGE PLANNING	Monitor progress on discharge plan; consult with MD, SW, and HHIC. MD to give 24 hrs. notice to patient and write official discharge order.	
PATIENT VARIANCE (On Admission)		

DATE	INITIALS	PRINT NAME	SIGNATURE

BETH ISRAEL MEDICAL CENTER
MULTI-DISCIPLINARY ACTION PLAN

DAY 3 OF 4

MD: _____

DIAGNOSIS: _____

DATE: _____

MAP DOES NOT REPLACE MD ORDERS

PATIENT PROBLEM	EXPECTED PATIENT OUTCOME/ DISCHARGE OUTCOME	NURSING INTERVENTIONS		ASSESSMENT/ INTERVENTION
1. Alteration in breathing pattern	1. Pt. will be free of respiratory distress as evidenced by: A. Resp. rate within normal limits for age. B. Arterial blood gases within normal limits. C. Equal air movement heard on ausculation. D. Clear breath sounds. E. Minimal work effort for breathing.	1A. Auscultate breath sounds, assess color, observe for retractions, nasal flaring every 8hrs. and PRN B. Vital signs with blood pressure, every 8hrs and PRN. C. Assess with MD readiness for change to po medications. D. Chest physical therapy every shift, unless contraindicated. E. Observe response to Nebulizer treatment and check with MD to decrease frequency. F. Peak flow every shift if >6 yrs. G. Assess pt's. response to activity H. Assess diet tolerance and record		
2. Knowledge deficit	2. The parent/child will verb. knowledge of teaching done regarding: A. Precipitating factors (Allergens, smoke, sudden changes in temp.). B. Meds, names, dose desired effects, adverse effects, frequency and times. C. Importance of regular follow-up appointments. D. Exercise regimen with breathing exercises.	2A. Continue ongoing discharge teaching i.e. medication administration, treatments, importance of follow-up. B. Disc. plan with parents to minimize allergies in the home. B₁ Reevaluate for VNS referral.		
3. Anxiety	3A. De-escalation of anxiety to within coping levels. B. Identify stress factors.	3A. Continue allowing verbalization of feelings, fears, and anxieties B. Provide emotional support. C. Reevaluate level of anxiety prn, provide supportive measures i.e. support groups OPD.		

BETH ISRAEL MEDICAL CENTER

MULTI-DISCIPLINARY ACTION PLAN

DAY 4 OF 4

MD: _____

DIAGNOSIS: _____

RN/MD REVIEW: _____

DATE: _____

MAP DOES NOT REPLACE MD ORDERS   **VARIANCE**

TESTS/ PROCEDURES/ TREATMENTS	Check theophylline level Peak flow every shift if >6yrs cooperative q8 hrs. Consider discharge if increased peak flow and improved clinical picture	
MEDICATIONS	Consider discharge home within 24 hours of initiation of po medication.	
ACTIVITY	As tolerated	
NUTRITION	As tolerated	
CONSULTS		
SOCIAL WORK	If patient is placed on ALC; all referral materials must be completed to CCMU within 24 hrs.	
DISCHARGE PLANNING	If patient is placed on ALC and is going to LTC faci- lity, transfer summaries must be completed prior to discharge. Prior to discharge confirm Home Care plans with SW and HHIC. Any patient with active CWA case must be cleared by social work.	
PATIENT VARIANCE (On Admission)		

DATE	INITIALS	PRINT NAME	SIGNATURE

BETH ISRAEL MEDICAL CENTER
MULTI-DISCIPLINARY ACTION PLAN

DAY 4 OF 4

MD: _____

DIAGNOSIS: _____

DATE: _____

MAP DOES NOT REPLACE MD ORDERS

PATIENT PROBLEM	EXPECTED PATIENT OUTCOME/ DISCHARGE OUTCOME	NURSING INTERVENTIONS		ASSESSMENT/ INTERVENTION
1. Alteration in breathing pattern	1. Pt. will be free of respiratory distress as evidenced by: A. Resp. rate within normal limits for age. B. Arterial blood gases within normal limits. C. Equal air movement heard on auscultation. D. Clear breath sounds. E. Minimal work effort for breathing.	1A. Auscultate breath sounds, assess color, observe for retractions, nasal flaring every 8hrs. and prn B. Vital signs with blood pressure, every 8hrs and PRN. C. Chest P.T. every shift, unless contraindicated. D. Observe response to Nebulizer treatment and check with MD to decrease frequency. E. Peak flow every shift if >6 yrs. F. Assess pt's. response to activity G. Assess diet tolerance and record. H. Assess clinical picture i.e. increased peak flow, toleration of PO meds., theophyline level between 10 & 20.		
2. Knowledge deficit	2. The parent/child will verb. knowledge of teaching done regarding: A. Precipitating factors (Allergens, smoke, sudden changes in temp.). B. Meds, names, dose desired effects, adverse effects, frequency and times. C. Importance of regular follow-up appointments. D. Exercise regimen with breathing exercises.	2A. Discharge Planning. B. Medications reviewed. C. Signs and symptoms of respiratory distress reviewed. D. Identification of factors that may precipitate asthmatic attacks. E. Exercise regimen, i.e. breathing exercises and rest periods. F. Follow-up care. G. When to call MD/come to E.R.		
3. Anxiety	3A. De-escalation of anxiety to within coping levels. B. Identify stress factors.	3A. Reevaluate level of anxiety and provide support prn. B. Reassure parents/child regarding knowledge of asthma.		

DATE/INITIALS	VARIANCE

DATE/INITIALS	VARIANCE

NRA 1175 REV 09/92

TUCSON MEDICAL CENTER
DIVISION OF NURSING
COLECTOMY
CarePlan MAP©

Developed by: Gail Greene, BSN, RN

NURSING DIAGNOSIS/ PATIENT PROBLEMS	OUTCOME EXPECTATIONS	EXPECTATIONS MET AT DISCHARGE Yes No Nurse's Signature
Pre-Operative		
A. Actual/potential for anxiety related to potential threat to well-being secondary to hospitalization and surgery.	A. Patient will express decreased amount of fear. B. Patient will identify any questions or concerns or needs necessary to decrease anxiety.	A. _____ _____ Date achieved: _____ B. _____ _____ Date achieved: _____
B. Actual/potential knowledge deficit related to surgery.	A. Patient will verbalize an understanding of nursing care. B. Patient will demonstrate compliance with nursing interventions.	A. _____ _____ Date achieved: _____ B. _____ _____ Date achieved: _____
Post-Operative		
1. Actual/potential for volume deficit related to NPO status, nausea and/or emesis.	Patient will obtain and maintain adequate hydration. A. Dressing is dry and intact.	A. _____ _____ Date achieved: _____

Continued.

NURSING DIAGNOSIS/ PATIENT PROBLEMS	OUTCOME EXPECTATIONS	EXPECTATIONS MET AT DISCHARGE Yes　No　Nurse's Signature
Post-Operative—cont'd		
	B. Heart rate within normal limits.	B. _____ Date achieved: _____
	C. B/P within normal limits.	C. _____ Date achieved: _____
	D. Mucosa pink and moist.	D. _____ Date achieved: _____
	E. Skin remains warm and dry without diaphoresis.	E. _____ Date achieved: _____
	F. Electrolyte balance at normal limits.	F. _____ Date achieved: _____
2. Actual/potential ineffective breathing pattern related to anesthesia and surgical pain.	Patient will maintain normal respiration pattern for patient.	_____ Date achieved: _____
3. Actual/potential for alteration in comfort: pain related to surgery.	A. Patient verbalizes absence or decrease in pain level. B. Participates in exercises and care.	A. _____ Date achieved: _____ B. _____ Date achieved: _____
	C. Comfortable and oriented to environment.	C. _____ Date achieved: _____
4. Actual/potential injury related to infection.	A. Skin integrity is maintained.	A. _____ Date achieved: _____

5. Actual/potential altered elimination: Constipation related to anesthesia, immobility, narcotics, and surgically changed pathway for stool.

B. Healing occurs without untoward evidence of infection, i.e., increased temperature, increased WBCs, wound redness, edema, or purulent drainage.

B. _____
Date achieved: _____

A. Patient will experience patient's normal bowel elimination pattern and will expel flatus.

A. _____
Date achieved: _____

B. Will be aware of and begin to understand changes regarding bowel function if ileostomy or colostomy are necessary.

B. _____
Date achieved: _____

6. Actual/potential altered elimination: Urinary retention related to anesthesia and surgery.

A. Patient will either:
• Urinate within 6 to 12 hours post surgery or 6 to 12 hours after catheter is discontinued.

A. _____
Date achieved: _____

• Pass 30 ml of urine per hour when patient has a catheter.

_____
Date achieved: _____

B. Will tolerate PO fluids without N/V prior to discontinuing IV fluids.

B. _____
Date achieved: _____

7. Actual/potential for injury.

Free of injuries during hospital stay.

_____
Date achieved: _____

8. Knowledge deficit as related to disease process and convalescent period.

Patient and significant others will verbalize acceptable level of knowledge and sign discharge instructions concerning:
A. Activity
B. Medication regimen

_____
Date achieved: _____

Continued.

NURSING DIAGNOSIS/ PATIENT PROBLEMS	OUTCOME EXPECTATIONS	EXPECTATIONS MET AT DISCHARGE Yes No Nurse's Signature
Post-Operative—cont'd	C. Future doctor appointment D. Diet E. Understanding symptoms requiring attention F. Hygiene changes relative to health status. G. Understand preprinted education materials regarding disease process. H. J.P. Tube care I. Other _____	
Additional Problems		
9. _____		_____ Date achieved: _____
10. _____		_____ Date achieved: _____

TUCSON MEDICAL CENTER
DIVISION OF NURSING
COLECTOMY
CarePlan MAP©

NRA 1175 REV 09/92   Developed by: Gail Greene, BSN, RN

PRE-OPERATIVE TEACHING—GUIDELINE AND DOCUMENTATION

Discuss the following with your patient and/or family before sending to surgery.

A. Pre-operative
    1. NPO means "Nothing by Mouth"
    2. Shower/pre-op
    3. Pre-op medication: Causes relaxation, dry mouth, drowsiness. Patient is to remain in bed after getting this medication.
    4. Transportation to holding areas.
    5. Disposition of valuables.
    6. Use of call bell systems.
    7. Turn, coughing, deep breathing.
    8. JP tube care

B. Intro-operative
    1. Recovery Room (PACU)—after surgery until awake and reacting (usually 1 to 2 hours)
    2. Frequent vital signs.
    3. Lots of people, no need for concern.

C. Post-operative
    1. Diet
    2. Activity
    3. Special checks or treatments
    4. Restriction, if any
    5. Exercises, breathing, extremities

Continued.

PRE-OPERATIVE TEACHING—GUIDELINE AND DOCUMENTATION—cont'd

6. Pain medicine—need to request
7. I.V.
8. Location after surgery
9. Voiding/catheterization
10. Possible tubes (i.e., foley, CT, NG, ET, invasive lines)
11. Possibility of colostomy or ileostomy

D. Fears, concern or other information requested: _____

_____

_____

E. Response to teaching: _____

F. Additional reinforcement needed on: _____

_____

_____

Nurse's Signature _____ Date _____

NRA 1175 REV 09/92

TUCSON MEDICAL CENTER
DIVISION OF NURSING
COLECTOMY
CarePlan MAP©

Developed by: Gail Greene, BSN, RN

INDEPENDENT ACTIONS BASED UPON THE HUMAN RESPONSE TO ACTUAL OR POTENTIAL PROBLEMS

Hospital Day	Consults	Tests	Activity/Rest	Medical Interventions	Medications	Nutrition	Nurses' Signatures
PTA or Day of Admit Date ____	-Anesthesia	-CBC -Urinalysis	-Up ad lib		-Own, if any	-NPO	_____
Surgery Date: ____		-Lytes if NG -H&H or CBC	-Up in PM to bathroom with help -If A-line; bedrest, turn, cough, & deep breath q 2 hours -Bed side commode with help	-IV -JP tube(s) -NG suction -Foley -Possible A-line	-Analgesics IM, IV, epidural -Antibiotics	-NPO, I&O	_____ _____ _____
Day 1 Date: ____		-Lytes if NG -H&H or CBC	-Walk in hall 4 times with assistance -If A-line: turn, cough, & deep breathe q 2 hours when in bed -Up in chair	-IV -JP tube(s) -NG to suction -Foley -A-line	-Analgesics IM, IV epidural -Antibiotics	-NPO, I&O	_____

All items not provided as planned. Enter explanation in the individualization/variance section on the last page.
DRG Number: 148/149. Expected LOS: 6-8 days.

TUCSON MEDICAL CENTER
DIVISION OF NURSING
COLECTOMY
CarePlan MAP©

NRA 1175 REV 09/92   Developed by: Gail Greene, BSN, RN

INDEPENDENT ACTIONS BASED UPON THE HUMAN RESPONSE TO ACTUAL OR POTENTIAL PROBLEMS

Hospital Day	Assessment	Discharge Planning	Teaching	Psycho Social	Self Care	Nurses' Signatures
PTA or Day of Admit Date: ___	-Lung status -Location and nature of pain		Reinforce pre-op teaching -Reassure and encourage patient that numerous people have ostomies and still enjoy active, happy and productive lives	-Assess anxiety level	-ADLs	___ ___ ___
Surgery Date: ___	-Lung status -Bowel sounds		-Reinforce post-teaching	-Continue to assess anxiety level -Inform of colostomy/ileostomy immediately post-op if one way constructed	-Assisted ADLs	___ ___ ___
Day 1 Date: ___	-Lung status -Bowel sounds	-Assess at home needs	-Continue to reinforce post-op teaching	-Continue to assess anxiety level -Patient to look at ostomy area during AM care and ostomy care. If no ostomy, look at incision area/dressing	-Assisted ADLs	___

All items not provided as planned. Enter explanation in the individualization/variance section on the last page.
DRG Number: 148/149. Expected LOS: 6-8 days.

TUCSON MEDICAL CENTER
DIVISION OF NURSING
COLECTOMY
CarePlan MAP©

NRA 1175 REV 09/92   Developed by: Gail Greene, BSN, RN

INDEPENDENT ACTIONS BASED UPON THE HUMAN RESPONSE TO ACTUAL OR POTENTIAL PROBLEMS

Hospital Day	Consults	Tests	Activity/Rest	Medical Interventions	Medications	Nutrition	Nurses' Signatures
Day 2 Date: ___	-If ordered, internist for resumption of usual meds	-Lytes if NG -H&H or CBC	-Walk in hall at least 4 times with help	-JP tube(s) -NG to suction -possible to go to clamping schedule, if ordered	-Analgesics PO -IM, IV, epidural, antibiotics	-NPO, I&O -Possible clear liquid (if ordered) -If total clamping scheduled (if ordered)	
Day 3 Date: ___			-Walk in hall at least 4 times with help	-Possible discontinue NG if ordered. Clamping schedule for NG if ordered -JP -IV	-IV, PO, IM, epidural. Antibiotics	-I&O -Clear liquid → full liquid late in day if tolerated clear liquids.	
Day 4 Date: ___			-Walk in hall at least 4 times (self ambulation)	-Possible Heparin well -JP tubes -Colostomy or ileostomy	-Analgesics PO or IM -Antibiotics	-Full liquid to diet as tolerated	

All items not provided as planned. Enter explanation in the individualization/variance section on the last page.
DRG Number: 148/149. Expected LOS: 6-8 days.

NRA-1175 REV 09/92

TUCSON MEDICAL CENTER
DIVISION OF NURSING
COLECTOMY
CarePlan MAP©

Developed by: Gail Greene, BSN, RN

INDEPENDENT ACTIONS BASED UPON THE HUMAN RESPONSE TO ACTUAL OR POTENTIAL PROBLEMS

Hospital Day	Assessment	Discharge Planning	Teaching	Psycho Social	Self Care	Nurses' Signatures
Day 2 Date: ___	-Lung status -Bowel sounds	-Assess at home needs -Ostomy to see patient if has ostomy.	-Continue to reinforce post-op teaching -Begin ostomy self-care teaching if has ostomy	-Continue to assess anxiety level -Begin handling ostomy equipment, possibly refer patient to ostomy client if available to decrease sense of isolation	-Assisted ADLs	___
Day 3 Date: ___	-Lung status -Bowel sounds	-Assess at home needs	-Continue to reinforce post-op & ostomy teaching -If path report indicates malignancy, give 1-800-4-CANCER number of patient access to more information	-Continue to assess anxiety level -Patient may choose to look at incision when dressing is changed -Empty own ostomy pouch	-Self ADLs	___
Day 4 Date: ___	-Lung status -Bowel sounds	-Assess at home needs	-Continue to reinforce post-op teaching -Continue ostomy teaching and assess patient response	Continue to assess anxiety level -Patient may choose to look at incision when dressing is changed -Empty own ostomy pouch	-Self ADLs	___

All items not provided as planned. Enter explanation in the individualization/variation section on the last page.
DRG Number: 148/149. Expected LOS: 6-8 days.

NRA-1175 REV 09/92

TUCSON MEDICAL CENTER
DIVISION OF NURSING
COLECTOMY
CarePlan MAP©

Developed by: Gail Greene, BSN, RN

INDEPENDENT ACTIONS BASED UPON THE HUMAN RESPONSE TO ACTUAL OR POTENTIAL PROBLEMS

Hospital Day	Consults	Tests	Activity/Rest	Medical Interventions	Medications	Nutrition	Nurses' Signatures
Day 5 Date:			-Walk in hall at least 4 times (self ambulation)	-Possible heparin line -JP tube(s) -Colostomy or ileostomy	-Analgesics PO -Antibiotics	Diet as tolerated	
Day 6 Date:				-Heparin line -Colostomy/ ileostomy			
Day 7 Date:							
Day 8 Date							

All items not provided as planned. Enter explanation in the individualization/variation section on the last page.
DRG Number: 148/149. Expected LOS: 6-8 days.

TUCSON MEDICAL CENTER
DIVISION OF NURSING
COLECTOMY
CarePlan MAP©

NRA 1175 REV 09/92

Developed by: Gail Greene, BSN, RN

INDEPENDENT ACTIONS BASED UPON THE HUMAN RESPONSE TO ACTUAL OR POTENTIAL PROBLEMS

Hospital Day	Assessment	Discharge Planning	Teaching	Psycho Social	Self Care	Nurses' Signatures
Day 5 Date: ___	-Lung status -Bowel sounds	-Assess at home needs -Continue Ostomy teaching and assess patient response	-Continue to reinforce post-op teaching	-Continue to assess anxiety level -Begin/continue self stoma care including changing bag, skin care as per ostomy if applicable	-Self ADLs	___ ___ ___
Day 6 Date: ___	-Lung status -Bowel sounds	-Assess at home needs -Continue Ostomy teaching and assess patient response	Ascertain that patient & family are competent to handle ostomy care (if applicable)	-Continue to assess anxiety level -Continue assisted/self stoma care if applicable	-Self ADLs	___ ___ ___
Day 7 Date: ___	-Lung status -Bowel sounds	-Assess at home needs -Continue Ostomy teaching and assess patient response	-Continue to assess for ostomy teaching	-Continue to assess anxiety level -Continue assisted/self stoma care if applicable	-Self ADLs	___ ___ ___
Day 8 Date: ___	-Lung status -Bowel sounds	-Assess at home needs -Continue Ostomy teaching and assess patient response	-Continue to assess for ostomy teaching -Review availability of Cancer Society as a resource if patient's surgery was due to a malignancy	-Continue to assess anxiety level -Continue assisted/self stoma care if applicable	-Self ADLs	___ ___ ___

All items not provided as planned. Enter explanation in the individualization/variance section on the last page.
DRG Number: 148/149. Expected LOS: 6-8 days.

NRA 1175 REV 09/92

TUCSON MEDICAL CENTER
DIVISION OF NURSING
COLECTOMY
CarePlan MAP©

Developed by: Gail Greene, BSN, RN

Date	Individualization/Variation	Cause	Action Taken	Signature

MAP Reviewed by:

Date: _____

Nurse Case Manager

Date: _____

Associate Case Manager

Date: _____

Associate Case Manager

Date: _____

All items not provided as planned. Enter explanation in the individualization/variance section on the last page.
DRG Number: 148/149. Expected LOS: 6-8 days.

MEDICAL REHABILITATION SERVICES
NURSING CRITICAL PATHWAY/CVA

St. Joseph Medical Center
3600 East Harry/Wichita, Kansas 67218/(316) 685-1111

Patient Name	Date of Admission
L or R CVA	Date of Discharge

ACTIVITY	DATE	VARIANCE
PREADMISSION		
• Introduction of patient/family to rehabilitation program		
• Give Stroke Packet		
Discuss Rehabilitation Concepts		
Clothing/laundry needs		
Conferences		
Family involvement		
Patient rights		
• Tour of department for family (patient if possible)		
• Introduction to Primary/Associate Nurse		
• Other _____		
ADMISSION DAY		
• Orientation to room		
Bedrails		
Call light system		
Emergency call system		
Bath/shower		
Toilet		
• Orientation to Rehab. 1A		
Dining room		
Therapies		
Library		
Conference room		
Other _____		
• Assess for prevention of falls		
• Rehab Nursing Admission Assessment completed in 8 hours		
• Identify problems and patient/family goals		
• Initiate Care Plan and complete Kardex		
• Identify patient/family educational needs		
• Other _____		
• List educational needs for Day 2		
Treatment Day 2		
• Educational needs		
_____		
_____		
_____		
• Review nursing assessment		

Continued.

ACTIVITY	DATE	VARIANCE
• Evaluate and update Care Plan and Kardex		
• Review and implement educational plan:		
Medications		
Elimination		
Skin		
Safety		
Other _____		
• Review Rehab. Nursing Care Plan/Goal with patient		
Set short term goals		
• Review Rehab. Nursing Care Plan/Goals with family		
Set short term goals		
• Alter nursing treatment plan, utilizing patient/family input		
• Nursing Care Plan completed		
• Patient/family signature on Care Plan		
• Other _____		
• List educational needs for Day 3		
Treatment Day 3		
• Educational needs		
_____		
_____		
_____		
• Review therapy goals		
• Incorporate support for therapy goals into Plan/Kardex		
• Review Nursing Care Plan		
• Initial Progress Note completed		
• Other _____		
• List educational needs for Day 4		
Treatment Day 4		
• Educational needs		
_____		
_____		
_____		
• Evaluate physical status:		
Medications/effects		
Weight		
Hydration		
Skin integrity		
Pressure areas		
Weight shifting		
Vital signs		
Other _____		
• Set long term goals with patient/family		
• Evaluate and update Care Plan and Kardex		
• Other _____		
• List educational needs for Day 5		

Continued.

ACTIVITY	DATE	VARIANCE
Treatment Day 5		
• Educational needs		
_____		
_____		
_____		
• Establish estimated length of stay		
• Verbal/written communication with case manager		
• Evaluate and update Care Plan and Kardex		
• Other _____		
• List educational needs for Days 6-7		
Treatment Days 6-7		
• Educational needs		
_____		
_____		
_____		
• Evaluate and update Care Plan and Kardex		
• Patient/family updated regarding plan		
• Introduce patient/family to library		
• Provide one educational opportunity in library		
• Other _____		
• List educational needs for Week Two		
WEEK TWO		
• Educational needs		
_____		
_____		
_____		

• Review/adjust B & B retraining program
  Patient is greater than 25% continent:
    Bladder   Yes/No
    Bowel Yes/No		

• Review and adjust safety needs		
• Review and set up support systems for therapy goals (Care Plan, Kardex, signage, etc.)		
• Weekly Progress Note completed		
• Evaluate and update Care Plan and Kardex		
• Patient/family updated regarding plan		
• Evaluate therapeutic day pass		
• Evaluate physical status:		
Medications/effects		
Weight		
Hydration		
Skin integrity		
Pressure areas		
Weight shifting		
Vital signs		
Other _____		
• Other _____		

Continued.

ACTIVITY	DATE	VARIANCE
• List educational needs for Week 3		
WEEK THREE		
• Educational needs		
_____		
_____		
_____		

• Review/adjust B & B retraining program
  Patient is greater than 50% continent:
    Bladder   Yes/No
    Bowel Yes/No		

• Review safety needs		
• Review and provide support systems for therapy goals		
• Weekly Progress Note completed		
• Evaluate and update Care Plan and Kardex		
• Patient/family updated regarding plan		
• Finalize continuing nursing recommendations		
• Community outing		
• Evaluate physical status:		
Medications/effects		
Weight		
Hydration		
Skin integrity		
Pressure areas		
Weight shifting		
Vital signs		
Other _____		
• Other _____		
• List educational needs to be completed and time frame		
LAST 4 DAYS		
• Completed educational needs:		
_____		
_____		
_____		
• Educational materials to be sent with patient:		
_____		
_____		

• Review B & B retraining program progress:
  Patient is continent of:
    Bladder   ____%
    Bowel ____%		

Followup plan includes:		
_____		
_____		
• Weekly Progress Note completed		
• Patient/family updated regarding plan		
• Discharge plan completed		
• Final instructions discussed with patient/family		

Continued.

ACTIVITY	DATE	VARIANCE
• Instructions documented		
• Following physicians notified of dismissal: _____ _____ _____		
• Prescriptions to patient/family		
• Other_____ _____ _____		

MEDICAL REHABILITATION SERVICES
PHYSICAL THERAPY CRITICAL PATHWAY/CVA

St. Joseph Medical Center
3600 East Harry/Wichita, Kansas 67218/(316) 685-1111

Patient Name	Date of Admission
L or R CVA	Date of Discharge

ACTIVITY	DATE	VARIANCE
WEEK ONE **Admission Day**		
• Introduction to patient/family and brief orientation to P.T.—if orders written by 1:00 pm. (N/A for Sunday/holiday admissions). Issue wheelchair and cushion, if appropriate.		
Treatment Day 2 Evaluation		
• Begin initial evaluation		
• Issue appropriate wheelchair and cushion, if not seen on Admission Day		
Treatment Day 3 Evaluation		
• Continue with evaluation		
• Instruct nursing and/or family in PROM to LE, if applicable		
• Document in Kardex the amount of assistance patient requires to do functional activities and issue appropriate equipment, if needed		
Treatment Day 4 Evaluation and Treatment		
• Complete evaluation		
• Set treatment goals/plan and discuss with patient/family		
• Initiate electrical stimulation program to shoulder, if subluxed		
Treatment Day 5 Treatment		
• Initiate treatment		
• Establish estimated length of stay		
• Written/verbal communication with case manager		
Weekend Days No OT, PT, Speech on Saturday or Sunday. Family Education Program available on Saturday mornings.		
WEEK TWO		
• Continue treatment and modify as needed		
• Determine need for Home Evaluation and complete. Copy to patient/family and case manager		
• Determine appropriateness for Community Outings		
• Initiate patient/family education—(i.e., bed mobility, transfers, wheelchair mobility, and car transfers, as appropriate)		
• Determine/order bracing, if needed		
• Evaluate therapeutic day pass, as appropriate		
WEEK THREE		
• Continue patient/family education (i.e., ambulation, floor transfers)		
• Finalize equipment recommendations by first of week		
• Finalize continued therapy recommendations		
• Community outing, if appropriate		
• Fit and train with orthosis, if applicable		
LAST 4 DAYS		
• Re-evaluation as indicated		
• Patient/family education completed		
• Home program completed, if indicated		

MEDICAL REHABILITATION SERVICES
OCCUPATIONAL THERAPY CRITICAL PATHWAY/CVA

St. Joseph Medical Center
3600 East Harry/Wichita, Kansas 67218/(316) 685-1111

Patient Name   Date of Admission
L or R CVA   Date of Discharge

ACTIVITY	DATE	VARIANCE
WEEK ONE **Admission Day** • Introduction to patient/family and brief orientation to O.T.—if orders written by 1:00 pm. (N/A for Sunday/holiday admissions).		
Treatment Day 2 Evaluation and Treatment • Evaluate ADLs		
• Evaluate and treat need for sling, lap tray, splints and other devices		
• Start evaluation of sensorimotor status		
Treatment Day 3 Evaluation and Treatment • Continue sensorimotor evaluation		
• Evaluate visual perceptual skills/cognition		
• Continue basic ADL evaluations		
Treatment Day 4 Evaluation and Treatment • Continue basic ADL evaluation		
• Continue visual perceptual skills/cognition evaluation		
• Set treatment goals/plan and discuss with patient/family		
Treatment Day 5 Treatment • Complete evaluations, if needed		
• Initiate treatment		
• Establish estimated length of stay		
• Written/verbal communication with case manager		
Weekend Days No OT, PT, Speech on Saturday or Sunday. Family Education Program available on Saturday mornings.		
WEEK TWO • Continue treatment and modify as needed		
• Determine need for Home Evaluation and complete. Copy to patient/family and case manager		
• Determine appropriateness for Community Outings		
• Initiate patient/family education—(i.e., SROM, toilet transfers, as appropriate)		
• Evaluate therapeutic day pass, as appropriate		
WEEK THREE • Continue patient/family education		
• Finalize equipment recommendations by first of week		
• Finalize continued therapy recommendations		
• Community outing, if appropriate		
• Evaluate homemaking skills, as needed		
• Evaluate complex ADLs, as needed		
LAST 4 DAYS • Re-evaluation as indicated		
• Patient/family education completed		
• Home program completed, if indicated		

MEDICAL REHABILITATION SERVICES
SPEECH THERAPY CRITICAL PATHWAY/CVA

St. Joseph Medical Center
3600 East Harry/Wichita, Kansas 67218/(316) 685-1111

Patient Name	Date of Admission
L or R CVA	Date of Discharge

ACTIVITY	DATE	VARIANCE
WEEK ONE		
Admission Day		
• Introduction to patient/family and brief orientation to Speech Therapy—if orders written by 1:00 pm. (N/A for Sunday/holiday admissions).		
Treatment Day 2		
• Assess swallowing, if ordered		
• Contact Physician or Physician's Assistant to make diet recommendations, if indicated		
• Post sign with diet/swallowing instructions in patient's room, if indicated		
• Discuss swallowing/diet recommendations with patient/family, if available		
• Discuss diet recommendations/special needs with nurse		
• Issue one-to-one communication device for amplification, if indicated		
• Determine need for modified barium swallow study		
• Initiate Speech/language evaluation		
Treatment Day 3		
• Continue Speech/Language evaluation		
Treatment Day 4		
• Continue evaluation		
• Set treatment goals/plan and discuss with patient/family		
Treatment Day 5		
• Initiate treatment		
• Continue in-depth evaluations, as indicated		
• Establish estimated length of stay		
• Written/verbal communication with case manager		
Weekend Days No OT, PT, Speech on Saturday or Sunday. Family Education Program available on Saturday mornings.		
WEEK TWO		
• Continue treatment and modify as needed		
• Re-assess swallowing/diet recommendations		
• Discuss updated recommendations regarding diet with nursing/patient/family		
• Determine appropriateness for Community Outings		
• Continue patient/family education regarding speech/voice/language/swallowing, as indicated		
• Evaluate therapeutic day pass, as appropriate		

Continued.

ACTIVITY	DATE	VARIANCE
WEEK THREE		
• Continue treatment and modify as needed		
• Re-assess swallowing/diet recommendations		
• Discuss updated recommendations regarding diet with nursing/ patient/family		
• Community outing, if appropriate		
• Finalize continued therapy recommendations		
• Continue patient/family education		
LAST 4 DAYS		
• Re-evaluation as indicated		
• Patient/family education completed		
• Home program completed, if indicated		

MEDICAL REHABILITATION SERVICES
CASE MANAGEMENT/SOCIAL WORK CRITICAL PATHWAY/CVA

 St. Joseph Medical Center
3600 East Harry/Wichita, Kansas 67218/(316) 685-1111

Patient Name	Date of Admission
L or R CVA	Date of Discharge

ACTIVITY	DATE	VARIANCE
WEEK ONE **First 48 Hours** • Initial contact made by SW/CM. Explanation of SW/CM roles, family conferences and discharge planning		
Within 72 Hours After Admission • Social history dictated		
Within First 7 Days • Initial family conference scheduled and communicated to patient and family		
• Evaluate discharge plan, financial resources and/or psychosocial concerns. Based on evaluation, action plan developed and implementation began (ongoing process)		
• Evaluate need for referral to Vocational Rehabilitation Services		
• Evaluate need for referral to Rehab Engineering		
WEEK TWO • Evaluate need for community resource referrals (ongoing)		
• Initiate and assist patient/family with application for financial assistance, if needed		
• Recertify with insurance company, if required		
WEEK THREE • Receive DME recommendations from team and evaluate insurance coverage for DME, if necessary		
• Obtain post-discharge therapy recommendations from team		
• Meet with patient/family regarding discharge plan, DME, and post-discharge therapy		
• Arrange acquisition of DME needs		
• Recertify with insurance company, if required		
• If extended care placement is recommended, evaluate availability and financial resources and communicate with family		
• Evaluate discharge transportation needs		
LAST 4 DAYS • Meet with patient/family to finalize discharge planning		
• Place Interagency and other communication forms on chart 48 hours prior to discharge		

MEDICAL REHABILITATION SERVICES
RECREATIONAL/ACTIVITY THERAPY CRITICAL PATHWAY/CVA

St. Joseph Medical Center
3600 East Harry/Wichita, Kansas 67218/(316) 685-1111

Patient Name	Date of Admission
L or R CVA	Date of Discharge

ACTIVITY	DATE	VARIANCE
WEEK ONE		
Admission Day		
• Introduction to patient/family and brief orientation to R.T./ Activities		
Treatment Day 2		
• Begin initial evaluation		
• Complete Leisure Interest Survey		
Treatment Day 3		
• Complete evaluation		
• Set treatment goals/plan and discuss with patient/family		
Treatment Day 4		
• Orientation to the available leisure programs, facilities and re- sources in the Medical Center		
• Encourage patient participation in scheduled weekly activities		
Treatment Day 5		
• Encourage patient participation in scheduled daily activities		
• Determine adaptations of activities to compensate for physical and/or cognitive limitations		
Weekend Days		
Encourage patient participation in scheduled activities/outings. Family Education Program available on Saturday mornings.		
WEEK TWO		
• Encourage patient participation in scheduled weekly activities		
• Determine appropriateness for community outings		
• Home evaluation, if appropriate		
• Continue patient/family education		
WEEK THREE		
• Encourage patient participation in scheduled weekly activities		
• Community outing, if appropriate		
• Provide information regarding community based support sys- tems		
• Provide information regarding appropriate community recre- ation resources		
LAST 4 DAYS		
• Re-evaluation as indicated		
• Patient/family education completed		
• Recommendations for post discharge/transition planning		

ST. MICHAEL HOSPITAL
MILWAUKEE, WISCONSIN

Uncomplicated MI Critical Path

DRG: _____

HCFA LOS: _____   Exp. LOS: _____

Physician: _____

Date Reviewed by Physician/RN: _____

Day/Date

	DAY 1 ED	DAY 1 CCU	DAY 2	DAY 3 Transfer to MCU	DAY 4
Floor:					
Consults:			Cardiac Rehab PT – – – – – and OT → Dietitian	– – – →	
Tests:	CBC EKG Lytes Glucose BUN Creatinine CXR Cardiac enzymes	CCU Standing Orders – – – → EKG – – – – – *Assess Need:* CPK Isoenzymes x 3 (total) per protocol Chem profile & elec- trolytes	EKG – – – – – Electrolytes in AM	EKG Stress test/cath ordered Day 7 or 8	EKG
Activity:	Bedrest – – – – –	– – – – – – – →	Bed rest c̄ commode PRN	Up in chair & progress – – → Progression of self-care ADL – →	
Treatments:	IV D$_5$W K̄o – – → Cardiovascular Assessment & VS q 10-15 min & PRN – – → Monitor – – –	Daily weights I&O VS q 4° & PRN	Heplock VI – VS q 8° & PRN	VS q 8° & PRN – – – – – – – – → – – – – – – – – – – – –	– – – – → – – – – – –

Continued.

Day/Date

Floor:	DAY 1 ED	DAY 1 CCU	DAY 2	DAY 3 Transfer to MCU	DAY 4
Medications:	Nitrates – – – – O_2 2-4 PNC – – – Analgesics – – – Lidocaine	$\longrightarrow$ – – – – – $\longrightarrow$ – – – – $\longrightarrow$ Stool softener Beta blockers Calcium channel blockers	O_2 PRN – $\longrightarrow$		
Diet:		Low cholesterol			
Discharge Planning:	Complete ED data base	Complete data base. Assessment of home situation	Mutual goal setting – – – $\longrightarrow$ *Multidisciplinary Staffing (T or F) Assessment of IP & OP plans of care. (*Inpatient Cardiac Rehab only)		Assess D/C needs & date Contact SW/HC prn

Key Nursing Diagnosis/Interventions:	-Orientation to ED, staff & equipment. *Assess & monitor:* -Head-to-toe assessment x 1 -Hemodynamic & cardiovascular stability (4) *Instruct:* -Pain scale 1-10 (1) -Preparation for adm. to CCU(2) [ ] brochure given [ ] family/sig. other notified -Offer emotional support	-Orientation to CCU routine, equipment, CCTV, & care delivery system. -Assess pain q 30" until under control (1) -Reinforce use of pain scale (1) -Position for comfort q 2° or prn (1) *Assess & Monitor:* -Head-to-toe assessment q 4° or prn -Activity restriction (3) -Hemodynamic & cardiovascular stability (4) -Arrhythmatic disturbances (4)	Position for comfort q 2° or prn (1) -Pt. booklet given (2) -Orient to CCTV, channels 3 & 11 (2) Review basic medication instruction c adm. of routine doses (2) *Instruct:* -ID risk factors specific c pt (2) -Diet modification (2) -Gradual progression of activity (3) – – –	Assess pt. readiness to learn, observe verbal/non-verbal cues, & pt's. condition (2) *Instruct: Stress Reduction (2)* -stress management relaxation techniques -time management -ID support systems & resources	– – – → → → → → → → →
Key Patient Activities/Outcomes:	-Pt &/or sig. other verbalizes fears & anxiety -Pt rates pain & intensity on 1-10 scale (1) – → -Pt. &/or sig. other verbalizes reason for hospitalization (2)	-Pt. demonstrates use of call light – → – – – → – – – → Pt's. behavior indicates pain reduction or elimination (1) Pt verbalizes that pain is decreased, alleviated, or under control (1)	-Pt. verbalizes understanding of diagnosis (2) -Pt. voices specific concerns related to coping with illness (2) -Pt. watches CCTV (2)	-Pt. behavior shows progress toward acceptance of illness (2) -Pt. able to identify own learning needs (2) -Pt. demonstrates readiness to learn (2) -Pt. verbalizes own risk factors (2) -Pt. demonstrates gradual progression of energy using energy conservation techniques (3&4)	– – → – – → – – → Behavior shows signs of: -stress management (2) -relaxation techniques (2) Pt. verbalizes time management skills (2&4) Pt. verbalizes support system & resources (2)

Continued.

Day/Date

	DAY 5	DAY 6	DAY 7-8	
Floor:	Transfer to 2N with telemetry			
Consults:		Assess Need OP Cardiac Rehab		
Tests:			Stress Test/Cath	
Activity:	Ambulate BID	Up ad lib		
Treatments:	VS q 8° & prn I&O	VS BID or q shift D/C I&O	D/C Heplock	
Medications:				
Diet:	Low cholesterol →			
Discharge Planning:		D/C orders D/C meds Follow-up MD appointment		
Key Nursing Diagnosis/ Interventions:	Review previous learning (2)	Review Home Program (2) -Post MI status -Diet -Meds a) schedule b) indications/side effects c) med sheet given -Follow-up with MD -Program given by pt.	OP Cardiac Rehab Post list	**Possible Nursing Diagnoses** 1) Pain 2) Knowledge deficit (Learning needs with diagnosis of MI) 3) Activity in tolerance 4) Decreased cardiac output *Nursing Care Guide available

| Key Patient Activities/ Outcomes: | Pt. verbalizes understanding of cardiac disease and/or MI (2) | Pt. plans activity progression and after D/C (home, work, sexuality, social) using energy conservation/work simplification techniques (2, 3, 4) | Pt. describes home med schedule with indications/side effects (reference med sheet) (2)

Pt. verbalizes follow-up MD, early warning signs, and emergency plan (2) | **WIPRO Criteria →**
All Met and Documented before Discharge
72 Hours a D/C
  No evidence of EKG changes.

48 Hours a D/C
  No change in type/dosage of antiarrhythmic drug(s).
  Chest pain controlled with anti-anginal drugs.
  Vital signs WNL for pt.

24 Hours a D/C
  Lab values WNL for pt. (lytes, BUN, enzymes)
  Oral temp <99°s antipyretic.
  Invasive monitoring devices removed.
  Activity/mobility/amb. documented as improved/ stabilized.
  Improved clinical status (e.g., chest clear, rales & wheezing, absence of friction rub & S, gallop).
  If DC'd to self care, document completion of pt. education.
  D/C plan documented.

If hospital stay < 3 days for R/O MI, no evidence of EKG changes or enzyme rise. |

Definitions

1. **DECREASED CARDIAC OUTPUT:**
   A state in which the blood pumped by the individual's heart is sufficiently reduced that it is inadequate to meet the needs of the body's tissues.

2. **PAIN:**
   A state in which an individual experiences and reports the presence of severe discomfort or an uncomfortable sensation.

3. **ACTIVITY INTOLERANCE:**
   A state in which an individual has insufficient physiological or psychological energy to endure or complete required or desired daily activities.

4/91 © St. Michael Hospital

Index

Custom Information You Need
From Mosby

THE NURSE MANAGER'S SURVIVAL GUIDE: PRACTICAL ANSWERS TO EVERYDAY PROBLEMS
T.M. Marrelli, RN, BSN, MA
1993 (0-8016-6449-7)

Finally, nurse managers have a resource for practical solutions to problems and challenges encountered daily. This quick-reference addresses crucial management activities, such as daily operations, time management, budgeting, and decision making. Nurse managers will also benefit from the book's coverage of key interpersonal management responsibilities, such as negotiating with others, handling patient and family complaints, delegating, motivating, and team building.

IMPLEMENTING SHARED GOVERNANCE: CREATING A PROFESSIONAL ORGANIZATION
Tim Porter-O'Grady, RN, EdD, CNAA
1993 (0-8016-6318-0)

This new resource provides an innovative and practical discussion of the most successful models of shared governance. Content focuses on the application of models in practice and presents well-structured and validated approaches to implementing shared governance.

Volume 5 in The Series on Nursing Administration
MANAGING NURSING CARE: PROMISE AND PITFALLS
Kathleen Kelly, RN, PhD
Meridean Maas, RN, PhD, FAAN
1993 (0-8016-6547-7)

With an emphasis on cost containment and quality management, this useful resource presents effective approaches to managing nursing care. The book describes specific models of case management and managed care in various settings— the community, HMOs, a hospital, and a long-term care facility. In addition, historical and future methods of managing care are explored. Analysis of education, research, and quality management issues related to managed care complete this thorough presentation.

To order call toll-free 800-426-4545. In Canada call 800-268-4178. We look forward to hearing from you soon!

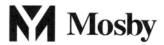 Mosby

NMA156

UNIVERSITY OF RHODE ISLAND LIBRARY

3 1222 00573 5876

DISCARDED
URI LIBRARY